I0786060

If you think you've read these blogs before, you're right. As I learned about writing and formatting my books of blogs, I realized *The Book of Blogs: Moderate Stage Chronic Kidney Disease, Parts 1 and 2* were unwieldy to hold and the type was too small, as well as having no index. I vowed to correct that. *Part 1* has already been separated into two books: *SlowItDownCKD 2011* and *SlowItDownCKD 2012*.

It seemed to take me forever to get to *Part 2* with life constantly getting in the way. Sure, a lot of that delay was for unwanted reasons like the medical conditions that were uncovered in my family and the deaths, but so much of it was good like the birth of my grandson, our travels, and the marriages of two of our daughters. Life is wonderfully complex that way.

The book series was begun after my family doctor told me I probably had a problem and it had to do with my kidneys, maybe Chronic Kidney Disease. My first reaction was to demand in no uncertain terms, "What Is It and How Did I Get It?" Hence, the title of my blog and the book with which the *SlowItDownCKD* series began.

There are many, many of us out there. By us, I mean those who have Chronic Kidney Disease. Friends, partners, family of CKD patients can all gain some insight into the daily travails of living with the disease via the blog and the books based on it, too. I am no expert, but I have read every book I could lay my hands on concerning this problem. Of course, most medical texts are not included because I couldn't understand them. Most of the kidney disease cookbooks aren't included because I can understand a heavy duty medical text better than I can a cookbook. I even read memoirs and biographies to glean what information I could.

Surprisingly, very few of these books dealt with the early or moderate stages of the disease. These are the stages when we, as patients, are most shocked, confused, depressed, and at sea. I didn't want to read about transplants or kidney failure. I just wasn't ready to learn about them. But I did want to know what was happening to me on a daily basis, what the medications that were ordered for me were supposed to do, and what new discoveries there were that might help slow down this deterioration of my kidneys. That's what the blog and the books are about.

The more you know about Chronic Kidney Disease and the more you read about other people's relationship with it, the more comfortable you'll feel in the early or moderate stages of having the disease yourself. I surely wish someone had blogged about it when it was new to me. As emails came in asking for print copies of the blogs for those who are not computer savvy or unable to gain access to a computer, I responded by publishing these books of blogs.

I've discovered I have something like 107,000 readers in 109 countries and they're not afraid to tell me what they need to know. I research for them and respond with a blog post, but remind them they need to speak with their nephrologist and/or renal nutritionist before taking any action since I am not a doctor.

I did write several previous books about Chronic Kidney Disease that you'll find referenced many times in the blogs. Those books are **What Is It and How Did I Get It? Early Stage Chronic Kidney Disease** and the other **SlowItDownCKD** titled books. Each in the series (except the first) consists of the blogs for one year. You can find them in print and digital on both Amazon.com and B&N.com. or you can walk into a Barnes and Noble to order them.

I began writing the blog after a doctor in India contacted me telling me he wanted his patients to have the first book, but sometimes they couldn't even afford the bus fare to the clinic. I suggested I start the blog (not having a clue how to do that), he translate it, then print it and give it to his patients. The idea was that those who could make it to the clinic would bring the printed copies of the blog back to their villages to share.

In the interest of keeping the book from becoming mammoth (again), I have omitted the blogs about websites, services, or products that are no longer available. Also omitted were sites that require membership and pay-for-use sites.

I've removed the pictures and a great many references to what was happening at that time in my personal life. I also removed my signature line: "Until next week, keep living your life!" After all, how many times can you read the same sentence in a single book?

When that still didn't shorten the books enough, I removed all notices of past book signings, book talks, Twitter chats, interviews, radio shows, and articles that I'd been involved with. You can't very well go back to the past, so why include them I reasoned.

When you see a set of braces rather than quotation marks, it's me inserting my thoughts into an article.

Welcome to **SlowItDownCKD 2014.**
Keep living your life,
Gail

p.s. As always, I want Bear to know how much I appreciate his respecting Monday as blog day, and when I'm writing a book, Monday, Tuesday, Wednesday, Thursday, Friday, Saturday, and Sunday as writing days. You're one of a kind, honey.

Book It!

1/5/14 With the holidays over and more time to think about what I'd like to write, I decided this would be a good time to update you about whatever other books are available that also concern Chronic Kidney Disease.

You know there are many out there, too many to mention here, so I eliminated any book that couldn't be understood by a lay person {Those without specific training in a certain field – in this case, medical} and renal diet books. You can easily find those for yourself by searching on Amazon.com and B&N.com. I also excluded those I found to be dubious… the spelling errors were a dead give-away that these were not professional.

Disclaimer: I am not a doctor, have never have claimed to be one, AND am not endorsing the following books, simply letting you know they exist. For the most part, the descriptions were written by the author, unless otherwise noted. The 'Look Inside!' function only works if you follow the link to Amazon.com – sorry!

I have been dreaming about this list, so let's get it out of my dreams and on the blog.

Ford, Mathea A., RD {Registered Dietician} ***Kidney Disease: Common Labs and Medical Terminology: The Patient's Perspective (Renal Diet HQ IQ Pre-Dialysis Living) (Volume 4)***
New to kidney failure? Have no idea what your physician just said about your kidneys? Kidney disease labs and terminology can quite often be a challenge to understand and digest. Did your doctor use the "stages of kidney disease"? Did you physician refer to "eGFR"? What does all this mean for your health and future with kidney disease, lifestyle and nutrition choices. This book is the basic platform for understanding all the common labs and terminology that your doctors and nurses will use. This book will give you and your caregivers the confidence to manage your condition knowing that you have an understanding of all the ins and outs of the nephrology jargon. {Mrs. Mathea seems to have an entire series of books about CKD.}

Hunt, Walter A. ***Kidney Disease: A Guide for Living***.
When Hunt learned he had kidney disease, he was overwhelmed by the prospect of facing kidney failure. He had so many questions: Why are my kidneys failing? Is there anything I can do to save them? How will I know when my kidneys have failed? What will it feel like? What treatments are available for me? Is there a cure for kidney failure? The good news, as Hunt found out, is that kidney failure is highly treatable. People with the disease can lead full and productive lives, and Hunt's readable and empathetic book will help them do just that. It discusses the latest scientific and medical findings about kidney disease, including what kidneys do; the underlying diseases that cause failure; diagnosis, treatment, and prevention; dietary factors; clinical trials; and the future direction of research on kidney failure. Kidney disease is difficult, but as Hunt's narrative reveals, people living with it can take control of their health and their future. By understanding kidney failure — what causes it, how it may affect their lives, and what treatment options they have — people with the disease can improve their quality of life and achieve the best possible outcome.

Lewis, Dr. Robert. ***Understanding Chronic Kidney Disease: A guide for the Non-Specialist***.
This is meant for primary care physicians, but can be easily understood by the layman. I looked under the covers of this one and was delighted to see that the information we, as patients with CKD, need to know is also what our primary care physicians need to know. {I wrote this description.}

National Kidney Foundation of Southern California. ***Living Well With Kidney Disease***.
The first edition of "Living Well With Kidney Disease" was developed and published by the National Kidney Foundation of Southern California. Based on the handbook "When Your Kidneys Fail" (originally published in 1982), this new and updated edition provides detailed information specifically intended for people coping with Kidney Disease and other renal failure, as well as their friends and families. The question and answer format provides a clear and manageable guide for those seeking support and answers. Among the topics covered are the principles of kidney function, methods of treatment, transplantation, and financial resources available to patients. With all of the ramifications of kidney

failure and the rise of Chronic Kidney Disease and Type 2 Diabetes, there is a growing population of people afflicted with kidney failure. Although it was written with the patient in mind, family members, friends and health care professionals will also find this handbook a valuable resource.

Synder, Rich DO {Doctor of Osteopathic Medicine} *What You Must Know About Kidney Disease: A Practical Guide to Using Conventional and Complementary Treatments*
The book is divided into three parts. Part One provides an overview of the kidneys' structure and function, as well as common kidney disorders. It also guides you in asking your doctor questions that will help you better understand both status and prognosis. Part Two examines kidney problems and their conventional treatments. Part Three provides an in depth look at the most effective complementary treatments, from lifestyle changes to alternative healing methods. The diagnosis of kidney disease is the first step of an unexpected journey.

It's always hard to find good books about CKD that non-medical personnel can understand. I hope these four and *What Is It and How Did I Get It? Early Stage Chronic Kidney Disease* help you feel more comfortable and knowledgeable about your diagnosis.

Just Breathe

1/13/14   Have I ever told you I have sleep apnea? And that this affects CKD patients? I do and it does. According one of the National Institutes of Health's sites, sleep apnea can raise blood pressure, which in itself is one of the problems of CKD. It can also result in glomerular hyper-filtration.

I wear something called a mandibular advancement device {MAD} while I sleep. I didn't want a Continuous Positive Airway Pressure machine, or CPAP as it is commonly called, because I don't like the idea of being tethered to anything – the same reason I am doing everything in my power NOT to get to the point when I need dialysis.

I didn't want surgery to correct the sleep apnea because of the drugs involved. I'm down to 48% kidney function, so I'd rather keep anything I haven't checked previously out of my body. Last time I had surgery, before the operation, I asked for and was given a list of the drugs to be used. I checked each with my nephrologist, but then – without advance warning – different drugs were used during surgery.

There's a little more than meets the eye to keeping your oral {Mouth} airways open at night. I love that play on words. Back to serious: the MAD forces your airway open by advancing your lower jaw or mandibular. A really nice by product is that you don't snore anymore, either.

A dentist who is a sleep apnea specialist needs to monitor your progress. When I first started, I was having so many episodes of sleep apnea {during which you stop breathing} that it was dangerous. And here I'd thought I was just a noisy sleeper.

This specialty dentist advanced the metal bars holding the top and bottom of the device together so that my lower jaw was moved further and further forward while I slept and my airway opened more and more.

While I am out of the danger range, I am still having those episodes of apnea so I keep driving from my home to Tempe {Between an hour and an hour and a half each way depending on the traffic} to have the device checked and adjusted every few months. This specialty dentist, the only one in the Valley of the Sun, then loans me a machine to measure the extent of my sleep apnea and the effectiveness of my MAD.

But that's not all. Since the mandibular is forced forward – good to open the airways, not so good for the muscles in the jaw – I also wear a retainer about half an hour after I remove, polish, and rinse the MAD. This retainer stays in my mouth for about 15 minutes, but I need to physically push the mandibular back in place so that my lower teeth can meet the retainer on my upper teeth. Result: I can't talk. Then this has to be brushed and dried, too.

In addition, I use a little machine that looks just like a jewelry cleaning machine in which I place a denture cleaning tablet once a week because there usually is some kind of buildup on the MAD.

This is quite a bit of work {adding to my daily routine of exercise, wearing hand braces at night, putting drops in my poor little macular degeneration suffering eyes... can I get a little sympathy here?}, but well worth it. I am not only saving my life, I'm saving my kidneys... and my heart... and my liver, according to the latest medical discoveries.

The down side? Well, if I open my mouth while I'm wearing the MAD, I drool. I could also risk stretching my jaw muscles if I don't use the morning retainer. Not using the retainer could result in a small, but permanent, shifting of my teeth as well. And there is pain when I first take out the MAD. Maybe I should write discomfort or minimal pain instead.

If you snore, get checked for sleep apnea. Many people just don't know they have it and, YES, it could be life threatening.

And Now for Something a Little Different

1/27/14 Just as with CKD, early detection of mesothelioma certainly helps in treating it. Screening the at risk population - those who have been exposed to asbestos - is an important part of detecting the disease, just as with CKD. However, there are reasons to be extra careful about diagnosing mesothelioma in kidney patients.

According to a September, 2011, study by PubMed, part of the US National Library of Medicine of The National Institutes of Health:

Serum mesothelin concentration is elevated in individuals with renal impairment. Renal function should therefore be taken into account during interpretation of this assay.

I wasn't clear about serum mesothelin so I researched it.

MedicineNet.com tells us that mesothelin is:

"A protein attached to the cell surface that is thought to have a role in cell-adhesion and possibly in cell-to-cell recognition and signaling. Mesothelin is so named because it is made by mesothelial cells. A monoclonal antibody, which recognises mesothelin, binds to the surface of cells from mesotheliomas and some other tumors but not to healthy tissues except for mesothelium."

So serum mesothelin is measured during a blood test. This tells your physician if you have mesothelioma and, if you do, how far it has progressed. BUT, if you have kidney disease, your readings for serum mesothelin may be elevated. What a Catch 22!

A little more on this. Serum means:

"The clear yellowish fluid obtained upon separating whole blood into its solid and liquid components after it has been allowed to clot."

This definition is from The Free Dictionary. You probably didn't need that defined, but I wanted you to see where in the blood you would find this indicator of mesothelioma. Notice that your creatinine measurement is also taken from the serum.

On another note, here's the first part of a blog by Dr. Robert Provenzano from *Accountable Kidney Care Collaborative* that resulted from the recent *Wall Street Journal* Article:

"The *Wall Street Journal* recently published an article about patients doing more to control chronic conditions. After finishing the article, my immediate thought was I'd like to see more patients like author Gail Rae-Garwood, who is profiled in the article, feel empowered to take charge of their health. Undoubtedly, patients need to muster a great deal of courage to step up and take the lead in managing their chronic kidney disease. And education is the best way for physicians to facilitate that kind of courage.

Educated patients make better clinical choices and are better prepared when treatment is necessary. This is a well-known fact, yet many patients need reinforcement to better understand how to live a longer, healthier, happier life—and that reinforcement can come from you, one of their most trusted resources."

I'm Tired.

2/3/14 I'm tired. I'm almost always tired. That is my most prevalent complaint lately. And Why? Because I have Chronic Kidney Disease, Stage 3A. I thought I remembered this particular symptom doesn't appear until dialysis starts – at stage 5 – so I decided to re-research my research... and surprised myself with the results.

I was becoming concerned. According to Donna D. Ignatavicius, MS RN, and M. Linda Workman, Ph.D, authors of *Medical-Surgical Nursing: Critical Thinking for Collaborative Care*, I shouldn't be. They explain that patients with early symptoms of chronic renal failure may complain of a general feeling of illness and that lack of energy and fatigue are often reported without any identifiable cause.

Okay, so maybe my CKD hadn't advanced and maybe I hadn't developed diabetes. Maybe it was just the stage of CKD I was in.

I wanted to check with my old standby, The Mayo Clinic. Their website told me:

Signs and symptoms of kidney disease may include:
- Nausea
- Vomiting
- Loss of appetite
- Fatigue and weakness
- Sleep problems
- Changes in urine output
- Decreased mental sharpness
- Muscle twitches and cramps
- Hiccups
- Swelling of feet and ankles
- Persistent itching
- Chest pain, if fluid builds up around the lining of the heart
- Shortness of breath, if fluid builds up in the lungs
- High blood pressure (hypertension) that's difficult to control

I also had never questioned why I have hiccups so often. Bear thought it was that I ate too fast, so I slowed down. {Hey, almost 45 years of running up to the fourth floor cafeteria, waiting in line, and then bolting down your food so you can get to the restroom and drop off your reports in the office three flights back down before teaching your next class doesn't dissipate that quickly. Long term habits...}

And why is fatigue a symptom of CKD in the first place? I found the following on KidneyABC.com.

Fatigue in CKD (Chronic Kidney Disease) is most often caused by anemia in which the count of red blood cells are {Sic} lower than normal. As red blood cells distribute oxygen to body tissues and cells, a shortage of oxygen can cause fatigue. Anemia begins in early stage of CKD, and tends to get worse as renal function decreases and less erythropoietin (EPO) is produced by kidneys.

This is something that I explained in *What Is It and How Did I Get It? Early Stage Chronic Kidney Disease.* I've been diagnosed with non-anemic low iron levels. Well, it's nice to know I'm not anemic, but the low levels of iron produce the same fatigue. Why?

The National Kidney and Urologic Diseases Information Clearinghouse explains.

Healthy kidneys produce a hormone called erythropoietin, or EPO, which stimulates the bone marrow to produce the proper number of red blood cells needed to carry oxygen to vital organs. Diseased kidneys, however, often don't make enough EPO. As a result, the bone marrow makes fewer red blood cells.

You can't correct it by simply taking EPO injections. It's just not that simple. To quote what I wrote in *What Is It and How Did I Get It? Early Stage Chronic Kidney*

...EPO can worsen your HBP – which can both cause and be caused by CKD. Most nephrologists agree it's better to take the EPO injections and increase your HBP medication to control your hypertension.

That was thought to be true when I researched for the book over three years ago, but since then the medical science community has discovered that synthetic EPO may be harmful to your body in that it may cause the body to produce antibodies for EOP. Then your liver becomes involved, too, since it produces a small amount of EPO.

So, what can you do for this fatigue? I went back to KidneyABC.com because their recommendations were simply so logical.

Regular exercises have many benefits for stage 3 CKD patients:
- Boost your energy.
- Improve your immune system.
- Alleviate edema.
- Lower high blood pressure.

Aerobic exercises such as walking, jogging, dancing, swimming, etc. are preferred. And remember to avoid strenuous exercises.

Sometimes I'm Down

2/10/14   My heart is heavy. That, of course, got me to wondering if this had anything to do with Chronic Kidney Disease. And it turns out, it does. While this sadness seems to always to be short term for me, it comes and goes for no apparent reason.

So I did what I do best. I researched... and found more than I'd expected about this subject.

Way back in 2009, The National Kidney Foundation, Inc. published their findings after performing a study:

Depression has long been associated with end stage kidney disease, but a new study published today in the *American Journal of Kidney Diseases,* the official journal of the National Kidney Foundation, found that 20% of patients with early stage Chronic Kidney Disease (CKD) also suffered from depression.

Looking further back, I noticed that in 2006, US National Library of Medicine, National Institutes of Health published a study on its PubMed site calling for:

...further well-designed, longitudinal, survival studies to clarify the relationship better between depression and the different stages of renal dysfunction.

So there is a connection. And I fell into that connection. Which doesn't mean that I'm clinically depressed or that I need treatment. What it does mean is that I need to accept that I will have my down days now and again... and they will pass.

Somehow, it strikes me that everyone – CKD patient or not – has such days.

DaVita has this to say about depression and CKD:

Depression can have many causes. In the case of someone who has just been diagnosed with Chronic Kidney Disease there may be a lot of information to process about your physical health, which may lead to strong emotions about your life and how it may change. Similarly, once a person reaches end stage renal disease and begins dialysis, there are lifestyle adjustments to be made that could bring up feelings of despair. Many times these feelings are temporary; however, if you find you're having difficulty don't hesitate to get the help you need.

It made sense to look at the other end and see if depression caused CKD, just as diabetes and/or high blood pressure may be both caused by CKD and may be the cause of CKD. The following is from a private mental health center in Scottsdale. It's especially interesting because of the size and duration of the study – 5,785 subjects under scrutiny for 10 years. It is also specific to CKD patients, although it is from 2010.

This particular study concluded that the patient population suffering from depression was more likely to develop kidney disease and a decline in kidney function. These studies are still in the very early stages and should not alarm anyone suffering from depression but should act as a motivator to encourage individuals to seek help for their depressive symptoms. On the other hand, it is known that depression is very common among patients with Chronic Kidney Disease and studies have shown that if the depression is left untreated, the prognosis of the kidney diseases is much worse.

Fresenius Medical Care, which is actually a dialysis provider, {No, I don't need dialysis; I just liked the comforting information on their site.} offers this distinction between common mood swings and depression:

You may already know that people with chronic diseases are even more prone to depression …. Depression is a broad term that describes a set of mood disorders. Some are long-term and some are short-term. Certain types are milder, while others are very strong and very harmful. For our purposes, we will place them into two groups: Common mood swings and Ongoing depression.

Everyone has common mood swings. They may look like depression, because you feel sad, discouraged, lack energy, may lose sleep, or doubt yourself over some event or relationship. These moods last from a few hours to a few days, and then subside. Clinically speaking, this is not depression, but a normal response to life changes.

It makes sense to list the symptoms of actual depression here so you can tell the difference between common mood swings and depression. *Make The Connection*, a veterans' support site tells us,

Not everyone with depression has the same symptoms or feels the same way. One person might have difficulty sitting still, while another may find it hard to get out of bed each day. Other symptoms that may be signs of depression or may go along with being depressed include:

- Feeling sad or hopeless
- Losing interest in or not getting pleasure from most of your daily activities
- Gaining or losing weight
- Eating more or less than usual almost every day
- Sleeping too much or not enough almost every day
- Feeling restless and unable to sit still
- Feeling that moving takes great effort
- Feeling tired or as if you have no energy almost every day
- Feeling unworthy or guilty nearly every day
- Having low self-esteem or feeling down on yourself
- Finding it hard to focus, remember things, or make decisions nearly every day
- Feeling anxious, worried, or nervous
- Drinking more alcohol or caffeine
- Taking more of a prescription or over-the-counter medication than as directed
- Smoking or using tobacco more often

You need to be careful. If you suspect you have depression, make sure you seek professional help. Not everyone gets to the point of feeling suicidal, but you want to make sure you don't.

The Dizzying Array of D Vitamins

2/17/14   Let's start at the beginning. What does vitamin D do for us? According to **What Is It and How Did I Get It? Early Stage Chronic Kidney Disease**, it

Regulates calcium and phosphorous blood levels as well as promoting bone formation, among other tasks – affects the immune system.

Short, sweet, and to the point.

But I think we need more here. Why are there different kinds of vitamin D? I went to Buzzle {My new favorite for easily understood renal information} and hit pay dirt on my first foray:

There are five different types of vitamin D. It seems to me that the source designates which number it is. For example, vitamin D2 comes from plants, small invertebrates, and funguses {Pay attention, vegans.} while the D3 that I take is manufactured synthetically. The designation D1 is no longer used, D4 is such a recent discovery that not much is known about it, and D5 is not technically a vitamin.

By the way, if your vitamin bottle doesn't have a number after the D, that means it's D2 or D3. You should know that the kidneys are responsible for transforming calcitriol into active vitamin D.

So, the sunshine vitamin is produced by our own bodies, but sometimes not at the rate we need it. Hence, we are prescribed vitamin supplements. As Chronic Kidney Disease patients, we need the extra vitamin D – whether from nature {D2} or synthetically produced {D3}. Why you ask? DaVita offers us this handy information.

Vitamin D	In CKD the kidney loses the ability to make vitamin D active. Supplementation with special active vitamin D is determined by calcium, phosphorus and PTH levels....	Helps the body absorb calcium and phosphorus; deposits these minerals in bones and teeth; regulates parathyroid hormone (PTH)

The site also suggests that vitamin D be by prescription only and closely monitored. Since it was my PCP who prescribed it for me {six years ago as a CKD patient}) and for Bear {last week and not a CKD patient}, I'm wondering if that caveat is for end stage Chronic Kidney Disease patients.

Notice we have a new term in the description above – parathyroid hormone. That's not as odd as it sounds. There is currently a controversy as to whether vitamin D is a vitamin or a hormone, since it is the only vitamin produced by the body. Here is an explanation of parathyroid hormone {PTH}.

The parathyroid glands are located in the neck, near or attached to the back side of the thyroid gland. Parathyroid hormone controls calcium, phosphorus, and vitamin D levels in the blood and bone.

Release of PTH is controlled by the level of calcium in the blood. Low blood calcium levels cause increased PTH to be released, while high blood calcium levels block PTH release.

And here you thought the kidneys worked alone to control these levels in the blood. Thanks to MedLine for correcting us. This National Institutes of Health site is a constant fount of pretty much any kind of health information you may need.

Okay, so let's say you don't take the vitamin D supplements you need. What happens to you then? I jumped right on to The Mayo Clinic site, but found their answer too general for my needs.

Vitamin D deficiency — when the level of vitamin D in your body is too low — can cause your bones to become thin, brittle or misshapen. The irony of this is that we live in the sunshine state. Only 20 minutes of sun a day could give us the vitamin D we need... and melanoma. Having had a brush with a precancerous growth already, I'm not willing to take the chance; hence, the supplements.

Let's not forget that vitamin D also helps absorb calcium and phosphorous, so it's not just your bones that are at stake, important as they are. I went back to the National Institutes of Health for more information. This is what they have to say.

Vitamin D is important to the body in many other ways as well. Muscles need it to move, for example, nerves need it to carry messages between the brain and every body part, and the immune system needs vitamin D to fight off invading bacteria and viruses.

Aha! Keep in mind that as CKD patients our immune systems are already compromised and you'll realize just how important this vitamin is to us.

Let's try it the other way. Let's say you are so gung ho on the benefits of vitamin D supplementation, that you take more than your doctor prescribed. Is that a problem? According to WebMD it is.

Too much vitamin D can cause an abnormally high blood calcium level, which could result in nausea, constipation, confusion, abnormal heart rhythm, and even kidney stones.

To sum up, you may be vitamin D deficient. Your blood tests will let you know. If it is recommended you take vitamin D supplements, stick to the prescribed dosage – no more, no less. While some foods like fatty fishes can offer you vitamin D, it's not really enough to make a difference.

I Feel Like a Heel

2/25/14 I do. And I have for months. But I didn't want to have this checked for months. I'm writing about what turned out to be plantar fasciitis, an inflammation of the connective tissue which supports the arch of the foot and is located between the heel and the ball of the foot. It is caused by small, repetitive trauma to this area. It almost sounds like carpal tunnel of the foot. I am being humorous here; don't take that seriously.

I had a referral for a podiatrist from my primary care doctor and I sat on it, until I realized that was what I was doing. I shook my head, took a deep breath, and made the call for an appointment. I'm glad I did. My fear had been that I would need surgery on the bone spurs in my heel. Plantar fasciitis has nothing, I repeat nothing, to do with the bone spurs in my case – although they can be a risk factor.

According to Beth Israel Deaconess Medical Center:

Plantar fasciitis is most common in people who are 40-60 years old. {How kind of my body to wait the extra seven years.} Other risk factors that increase your chance of getting plantar fasciitis include

- Physical exertion, especially in sports such as:
  Running
  Volleyball
  Tennis
- A sudden increase in exercise intensity or duration
- Physical activity that stresses the plantar fascia
- People who spend a lot of time standing
- A sudden increase in activities that affect the feet
- Obesity or weight gain {Ummm}
- Pre-existing foot problems, including an abnormally tight Achilles tendon, flat feet, or an ankle that rolls inward too much
- Poor footwear {Ack! Grew up with that and overcompensated with exactly the wrong kind of shoes as an adult.}
- Heel spurs {Luckily for me, not in my case}

The podiatrists I chose are treating it with rest – one of the hardest things for me to do, even in my 'retirement.' When I explained that I needed to exercise at least half an hour daily for the Chronic Kidney Disease, they amended that to using the stationary bike {Well, they gave me a handout that included cross-training. I wasn't sure what that was, but I'm good at asking.} It almost felt good to get back on the bike this morning.

They also suggested swimming, certain kinds of yoga, and certain kinds of weight training. I'll stick with the stationary bike, thanks.

But that, of course, is not all. I already messed this one up by misreading, but I'll do it right tonight! I'm to freeze a sports bottle {still not sure how that's different from a regular bottle.} and roll it over my arch for 20 minutes every evening. Not bad, I can read while I do that… I think.

I also need to stretch my calf multiple times a day. That's not hard to do. Remembering to do it is the hard part.

Here's the kicker {Ouch!} - I have to wear shoes that meet the following criteria.
- A firm heel counter. {I had to ask look that up. I found this definition at shoesglossary.com: A piece of leather forming the back of a shoe or boot. A heel counter may be used to stiffen the material around the heel and to give support to the foot. }
- A rigid shank {the part of the shoe between the inner and outer soles}.
- A flexible toe.

World Kidney Day

3/10/14   Thursday, March 13th, is World Kidney Day. It's always the second Thursday in March. But what is it? And who started it? And why? I discovered this is a fairly new designation. It was only eight years ago that it was initiated.

According to World Kidney Day:

World Kidney Day aims to raise awareness of the importance of our kidneys to our overall health and to reduce the frequency and impact of kidney disease and its associated health problems worldwide.

The 54 year old International Society of Nephrology {ISN} – a non-profit group spreading over 126 countries – is one part of the equation for their success. Another is the 15 year old International Federation of Kidney Foundations. Add to that The World Kidney Day Team and you have the makings of this particular concept.

While 157 countries celebrated last year, I suspect this year even more countries will be involved. Why, you ask? This year's theme is Chronic Kidney Disease and Aging. We all age... in every country... in every part of the world... whether we've been diagnosed with CKD or not.

While there are numerous objectives for this year's World Kidney Day, the one that lays closest to my heart is this one:

Educate all medical professionals about their key role in detecting and reducing the risk of CKD, particularly in high risk populations.

Their site offers materials and ideas for celebrations as well as a page to post your own activity. Take a look at the map of global celebrations and prepare to be awed at how wide spread World Kidney Day celebrations are.

Before you leave their page, take a detour to Kidney FAQ {Frequently Asked Questions} on the toolbar at the top of the page. You can learn everything you need to know from what the kidneys do to what the symptoms {or lack thereof} of CKD are, from how to treat CKD to what to ask your doctor, plus a toolbox full of helpful education from about your kidneys to preventative measures.

For those of you who have forgotten, easily read explanations of what results of the different items on your tests mean are in ***What Is It and How Did I Get It? Early Stage Chronic Kidney Disease***; all it takes is a blood test and a urine test. I have routine blood tests every three months to monitor a medication I'm taking. It was in this test, a test I took anyway, that my family physician uncovered Chronic Kidney Disease as a problem.

Oh, By The Way….

3/17/14 In honor of National Kidney Month, I asked my daughter Nima Beckie {blogger extraordinaire at *Is What It Is*} to guest blog explaining what it's like to be the grown child of a Chronic Kidney Disease patient. I think she's outdone herself {Of course, I might just be a smidgen prejudiced, but I don't think so.}

■■

Several years ago my mom, Gail Rae-Garwood, came to us all and told us she'd been diagnosed with Chronic Kidney Disease. At the time none of us had the first clue what that meant (Actually, at the time I might have thought it was a distant cousin of an EKG.) and couldn't quite put two and two together.

I'm caring by nature and want to help, almost to the point where it can become overbearing. From my uneducated fear came wanting to make sure my mother was getting enough rest if we were out when I was visiting and asking all the time, "Have you had enough? Do you need a rest?"

If you're an adult child with parents who have kidney disease… DON'T DO THIS!!! What I learned along the way is that while your parents and loved ones truly appreciate your care and concern, they don't want you babying, coddling, or suffocating them.

Here's what you CAN do instead. Ask questions and educate yourself. Get involved in the kidney community when you can. Show your support that way.

I got involved because my mother wrote **What Is It and How Did I Get It? Early Stage Chronic Kidney Disease**. I helped out by acting as a reader for her, and then helping her approach the somewhat awkward (for her) task of Social Media.

The more I went back and read her blog, or helped out with Facebook, or Twitter, or read chapters of the book, the more educated about Chronic Kidney Disease I became.

I know that too much information thrown at you once can be like

"Whoa?! What?!" Honestly, I still refer to the blood test I get to check for kidney disease as a BUN (the kind you eat) as opposed to a B.U.N., and am still not in the least bit fluent in medicalese.

Last October, I took a big step—actually about eight miles worth of them. It was important to me to not just be an activist for the kidney community online, but in person as well.

I made my way to Foley Square in New York City near where I live (close to my Mom's hometown), donned an orange tee-shirt, and spent my morning volunteering for the GNYKF (Greater New York Kidney Foundation).

I helped others who were there to walk sign the banner that would be carried in front of the walkers. I'd ask each person, "Why are you here?" "Who are you walking for today?" So many faces, and so many stories and there isn't one that didn't touch my heart.

A lot of people were there for their family members, some who sadly didn't make it. One was a dad whose 12 year old son was waiting for his second transplant, as the first one didn't take. He was so proud of his son, but you could see the fear and hurt for his son in his eyes.

Another woman looked at me, and said, "I'm here because I'm waiting for a kidney. Is that a good enough reason?" I quickly walked around to the other side of the table to give her a big hug. I told her, just like I'm telling all of you, "I want you to know you are my hero. I know how hard you fight every day, and I know it's not always easy. I see you." She said her husband told her that all the time, and she never believed him.

Another little girl was there because a girl in her class "...was sick with kidney disease" and she wanted to help her. I asked her if she knew where her kidneys were... (sort of...). I showed her, and told her, "You are doing an awesome thing for your friend and should be so proud of yourself." Then I made her give herself a pat on the back (and may have whispered to her mom that there was a face painting table in the corner)

Lastly, I walked with so many people all wearing orange all the way over the Brooklyn Bridge and back – all in support of the same cause, all hoping for a cure. On the way back, I managed to snap a picture of a man taking his orange bandana from his head, and tying it at the halfway point of the Brooklyn Bridge for people fighting kidney disease everywhere.

There really are no words for moments like that. I'd worn the bracelet my mom bought for me not long after she'd moved to Glendale so she'd be with me. As I got to the finish line, the song "New York State of Mind" by Alicia Keys was playing, which was just so perfect, since I was walking for my mom in her home state. I crossed under the balloons, and called my mom.

She couldn't pick up because she was having a bad day. Severe bronchitis from a weakened immune system. I left a voicemail, "I want you to know, this is for you. I see everything you do. I know how hard you work, even on days when it isn't always easy, because you don't feel well. I know how much you help people. You are and forever will be my hero. I love you." I'll let her tell you what she said in response...I still have it saved on my phone.

Here's my last piece of advice, and it's a biggie. Get yourself tested. Every time you go to a doctor, it's up to you to mention to your doctor, "Oh by the way...I have a family member that has kidney disease," and request both your B.U.N and creatinine levels. This is simple blood work that takes two seconds but, in the end, could save you a lot of heartache.

Actually, I want to take that back a second, EVEN IF YOU DON'T have a family member with kidney disease, you should be getting checked regularly and educating yourself.

More than half the population in this country is at risk for kidney disease and many of them don't know it. That's an awfully big number, and it doesn't need to be. A smart lady who you may know raised me to believe that knowledge is power. Educate yourselves, educate your friends, and get tested...Happy National Kidney Month!!

It's Still National Kidney Month

3/24/14   And I still have pre diabetes. It sounds like something someone made up and maybe it is, but my A1C test result is still high and getting higher despite the changes I've made in my eating habits. When better than National Kidney Month to explain why this could be a problem for those of us with Chronic Kidney Disease?

We'll need a little background here, as usual. First, what is the A1C test? According to The Mayo Clinic:

The A1C test result reflects your average blood sugar level for the past two to three months. Specifically, the A1C test measures what percentage of your hemoglobin — a protein in red blood cells that carries oxygen — is coated with sugar (glycated). The higher your A1C level, the poorer your blood sugar control and the higher your risk of diabetes complications.

I'm sure you noticed how often I rely on The Mayo Clinic for definitions. I find their simple explanations make it easier for me {and my readers} to understand the material. I also like that they explain in their explanations. These phrases surrounded by dashes or in parentheses further clarify whatever the new term may be.

Okay, so we can see why this needs to be tested. Now, what does it have to do with diabetes and what is diabetes anyway? This time I looked for a medical dictionary and found one at our old friend, The Free Dictionary. The mellitus is there because that's how members of the medical field usually refer to diabetes – as diabetes mellitus. This is what I found there.

Diabetes mellitus is a condition in which the pancreas no longer produces enough insulin or cells stop responding to the insulin that is produced, so that glucose in the blood cannot be absorbed into the cells of the body. Symptoms include frequent urination, lethargy, excessive thirst, and hunger. The treatment includes changes in diet, oral medications, and in some cases, daily injections of insulin.

In **What Is It and How Did I Get It? Early Stage Chronic Kidney Disease** I define glucose as the main sugar found in the blood. I go on to explain that in diabetes, the body doesn't adequately control natural and ingested sugar. The Free Dictionary definition shows us how the body loses control of insulin production and what it means for the glucose levels... which is what the A1C test measures.

So... PRE diabetes? What's that? Funny you should ask. The English teacher in me can tell you that pre is a prefix {a group of letters added at the beginning of a word that changes its definition} meaning before. Pre diabetes literally means before diabetes which makes no sense to me because that would mean everyone without diabetes was pre diabetic. It helped me understand when I was told pre diabetes was formerly called borderline diabetes, a much better term for it in my way of thinking.

This time I went to WebMD for a simple explanation. In addition to learning that pre diabetes means your glucose, while not diabetic, is higher than normal, I found this interesting statement:

When glucose builds up in the blood, it can damage the tiny blood vessels in the kidneys, heart, eyes, and nervous system.

KIDNEYS!

Well, then what's a normal level you ask? According to my primary care physician, 4.8-6.0 is normal BUT this range needs to be adjusted for Chronic Kidney Disease patients. I looked this up at Lab Tests Online and found more of a range.

- A nondiabetic person will have an A1C result less than 5.7%.
- Diabetes: A1C level is 6.5% or higher.
- Increased risk of developing diabetes in the future: A1C of 5.7% to 6.4%

My result was 6 in the emergency room last November. During my regularly scheduled CKD yearly lab last September, it was 5.9 with a big H for high next to it. The August before that it had been 6.1. Back in January of last year, it was 6. I seem to be staying in a very close range for over a year, but it's still pre diabetes.

All right then, what's normal for a CKD patient? I don't know. Life Options says just keep it under 6.5. The rest of the internet seems to think the A1C results need to be adjusted only if you have both diabetes and CKD. Looks like my nephrologist and I will have to have another talk about this.

You would think the danger of an elevated A1C would be diabetes, but I'm wondering if the damage to those tiny blood vessels may be worse. Have I raised questions in your mind? Is your A1C normal? How do you tell if different sources hold different values as normal? Time to ask your doctor. And time to remind you again, that I am NOT a doctor, just a CKD patient with loads of questions and a willingness to research some answers for us all. Something to consider.

Other things to consider: have you had your kidneys tested? It's a simple blood test and a simple urine test. Sure you don't have the time, but no one does. Then again, it's sure worth it to avoid the need for dialysis {Now THAT takes time.} and a transplant down the road.
You know that 59% of our country's population is at risk for CKD, but did you know that 13 million U.S. citizens have undiagnosed CKD? That's scary. Take the test.

Good bye to National Kidney Month

3/31/14 Facts from the National Institutes of Health.

- Cardiovascular disease is the main cause of death in dialysis patients.
- Medicare is spending 6% of its payouts on kidney care.
- Kidney disease runs in families.

Of course, now you're thoroughly grossed out and maybe scared out of your mind about CKD. Good! That's exactly what I was aiming for. I don't see the point in you, your best buddy, your child, anyone who touches your life being diagnosed at stage 3 as I was. I wasted all of stage 1 and stage 2 when I could have been spending that time working to SLOW the decline of my kidneys so I could be one of the 80% of CKD patients who never needs dialysis or a transplant {And, no, I don't mean because I already died}.

And why did I waste that much time instead of prolonging my life? I was never tested. That's it. Simple, direct, and to the point. The fear here should be in having CKD and not knowing it instead of fearing you have it. If it turns out you don't have CKD, I am extremely happy for you and maybe a bit envious. But if you do, let's start working on prolonging your life NOW. You realize I'm not talking about a year or two, but decades here.

The tests themselves are simple. Do you urinate? {You'd better be responding in the positive here or you've already got a bigger problem than CKD.} Then you can just urinate into a vial instead of the toilet. No special training needed.

Ever have your blood drawn? Did you die from it? { know, I know, but it's a rhetorical question.} Okay, so have your blood drawn again and ask to be tested for Chronic Kidney Disease. It is not a separate blood test, but can be included in one you may be having anyway.

So it's goodbye to National Kidney Month, but not to taking care of yourself... say good bye by having the blood and urine tests for CKD. Be a pal. If you can't do it for yourself, do it for me. Don't deprive the world of the pleasure of your company because you didn't take the test.

Happy Anniversary... Sort Of

4/7/14   Yesterday was our first anniversary. We were glad to start Year Two as a married couple, but not before we celebrated the end of the first year by eating the piece of wedding cake our well-meaning friends had insisted be placed in an airtight plastic bag and frozen for a year.

Of course, that meant to me that we should have the special ground coffee I had ordered for the wedding with the cake, so I saved some of that, too. My daughter, Nima, had been a Starbuck's barista for a time and carefully explained to me that you don't freeze or refrigerate coffee. So I just folded over the top of the bag and clipped it shut.

Hang on and you'll eventually see what the wedding cake tradition and the coffee have to do with CKD. Back to the cake: I scouted around and found this freezing guide at Home Storage Solutions 101.

Bread & Desserts	Time
Baked bread and cookies	3 months
Cakes, pastries and doughnuts	3 months
Muffins and quick breads	3 months
Pancakes and waffles	3 months
Cooke or bread dough	1 month

Produce	Time
Fruits	1 year
Juices	1 year
Vegetables	8 months
Nuts	3 months

Dairy & Eggs	Time
Ice cream	2 months
Butter	9 months
Cheese	3 months
Eggs (raw, not in shells)	1 year
Milk	1 month

Meats	**TIme**
Ground beef, pork & stew meats	4 months
Other beef (i.e., roasts, steaks)	1 year
Lamb and veal	9 months
Ham	2 months
Pork chops	4 months
Pork roast or loin	8 months
Bacon and sausage	1 month

Poultry	**TIme**
Chicken and turkey (whole)	1 year
Chicken and turkey (cuts)	6 months
Ground turkey and chicken	4 months

Seafood	**TIme**
Fatty fish (i.e., mackerel, trout)	3 months
Lean fish (i.e., cod, flounder)	6 months
Crab	10 months
Lobster	1 year
Shrimp and scallops (unbreaded)	1 year

Miscellaneous	**TIme**
Casseroles (cooked)	3 months
Paste and rice (cooked)	3 months
Soups and stews	2 months

This is not the gospel of freezing food, but I wanted to give you a general guideline. Did you notice that "3 months" for cakes? I think I'm beginning to understand the stomach ailment now. {She groaned.}

That, of course, made me wonder how long ground coffee could keep if it wasn't frozen or refrigerated, which would have made it take on the taste of its neighbors and help destroy its own wonderful flavor. I went to Eat By Date for this chart.

(Unopened/Sealed)	Pantry	Freezer
Ground Coffee lasts for	3-5 Months	1-2 Years
Whole Bean Coffee lasts for	6-9 Months	2-3 Years
Instant Coffee lasts for	2-20 Years	Indefinite

(Opened)	Pantry	Freezer
Ground Coffee lasts for	3-5 Months	3-5 Months
Coffee Beans last for	6 Months	2 Years
Instant Coffee (freeze dried)lasts for	2-20 Years	Indefinite

Ugh! A year is substantially more than the 3 to 5 months suggested. Okay, so now you have the back story.

Thanks for being patient. Here's where the CKD comes in. Your kidneys filter toxins and waste products from your blood. They also regulate electrolyte levels and blood pressure and produce hormones, among their many jobs. If they're busy taking care of food poisoning {Or whatever you call eating improperly or overly frozen or stored food}, they have less time – or is it energy? – to pay attention to their typical jobs. There's even a theory that food poisoning can further compromise our already compromised immune systems.

It's the Salt of the Earth

4/14/14 A friend's not using salt in her cooking got me to thinking if we needed salt at all. Actually, I knew we did, but I didn't know why. I poked around and found the following on an NPR blog.

"If you don't keep up your sodium level in your body, you will die," explains Paul Breslin, a researcher at **the** Monell Center, a research institute in downtown Philadelphia devoted to the senses of taste and smell.

That's extraordinarily blunt. What I got from this is the same question I usually have: why?

I remembered that salt regulates your hydration but decided to check this anyway. According to The Royal Academy of Chemistry
It is the sodium (ions) present in salt that the body requires in order to perform a variety of essential functions. Salt helps maintain the fluid in our blood cells and is used to transmit information in our nerves and muscles. It is also used in the uptake of certain nutrients from our small intestines. The body cannot make salt and so we are reliant on food to ensure that we get the required intake.

Erukalert.org made me realize another important function of sodium, the element our bodies cannot produce:

Researchers at McGill University have found that sodium – the main chemical component in table salt – is a unique "on/off" switch for a major neurotransmitter receptor in the brain. This receptor, known as the kainate receptor, is fundamental for normal brain function and is implicated in numerous diseases, such as epilepsy neuropathic pain.

Normal brain function!

Just in case you didn't take chemistry in high school or college – which I admit was too intimidating for me – salt is 40% sodium and 60% chloride. It's the 40% sodium that causes a problem if you have too much of it. This is a quandary. You need salt to live and function well, but too much can kill you via raising your blood pressure.

There is an ongoing controversy of how much salt we need on a daily basis. This is what is on Colorado State's website {the academic institution}:

The Dietary Guidelines for Americans recommended reducing sodium intake to no more than 2,300 milligrams per day. However, those with hypertension, over the age of 51, or who are African American, should consume no more than 1,500 milligrams of sodium per day. This recommendation includes over half of all Americans.

But have they taken into account the fact that we sweat during the summer or when we work out and lose a great deal of sodium that way? Does that mean we need more sodium during these times? And how do you judge how much sodium is too much anyway? Or do we use the Goldilocks Theory of 'just right' here.

All right, then. The next logical question would be how much is usually too much. Hello, Medical News Today. That's where I found this handy, dandy, how much chart:

You should learn how to read food labels and identify high and low salt foods. You should check the labels of foods to find out which ones are high and low in salt content. If the label has more than 1.5g of salt (or 0.6g of sodium) per 100g it is a high salt content food. If it has 0.3g of salt (0.1g of sodium) per 100g then it is a low salt content food. Anything in between is a medium salt content food.

- **High** salt content food = 1.5g of salt (or 0.6g of sodium) per 100g
- **Medium** salt content food = between the High and Low figures
- **Low** salt content food = 0.3g of salt (0.1g of sodium) per 100g

The amount you eat of a particular food decides how much salt you will get from it.

As renal patients, we need to pay special attention to the amount of sodium we ingest. I'm on the Northern Arizona Council of Renal Dietitians' diet which permits 2,000 mg. of sodium a day. That's really limited since a teaspoon of salt has about 2,300 mg. of sodium. Of course, now that I'm over 51 {okay, way over}, I'm down to 1,500 mg. of sodium daily.

How do I keep within my guidelines, you ask? It's become easy, but don't forget I've had seven years to perfect it. We do have filled salt shakers available in the kitchen, but they're invisible to me. I use spices in cooking instead. My best friend there is Mrs. Dash's, although there are many other spices on the renal diet. I just like her blends. I check labels copiously when I do the marketing and Bear does too. If there's hidden sodium in foods, there's not much I can do about it. However, checking labels and ignoring the salt shaker will help keep my kidneys safe from too much sodium. {Pssst: I also ignore whatever food you can buy at gas stations.}

As DaVita tells us:

Particularly damaging is sodium's link to high blood pressure. High blood pressure can cause more damage to unhealthy kidneys. This damage further reduces kidney function, resulting in even more fluid and waste build up in the body.

Other sodium-related complications include the following:

1. Edema: noticeable swelling in your legs, hands and face
2. Heart failure: excess fluid in the bloodstream can overwork your heart making it enlarged and weak
3. Shortness of breath: fluid can build up in the lungs, making it difficult to breathe.

Another Holiday

4/21/14   What a relief to find I could cook for the holidays without too much referring to the renal diet bible. It took almost seven years for this information and this way of being to become part of me. The point here is that the renal diet has become a way of life, one I don't often think about too much anymore. I can easily remember a time I needed to pull out the diet list to see what I could eat, then another list to see if the protein, potassium, phosphorous, or sodium {3 Ps and an S, as I call them in ***What Is It and How Did I Get It? Early Stage Chronic Kidney Disease***} levels were too high, and finally the KidneyDiet app to make sure I hadn't gone over my limits for each of these and a calorie count.

This wonderful revelation doesn't mean that I don't hit my own 'refresh' button periodically to make sure I really am correctly eye judging the amounts of each food I use in cooking and eating or that I don't need to occasionally check to see if I'm right about the amount of whatever is in it.

I still carry all three of these – Northern Arizona Council on Renal Nutrition Diet, AAKP Nutrition Counter, and KidneyDiet app – as my talismen. There's a certain security in knowing I have them if I need them. I also find that sometimes I just don't remember exactly what I read in each, so it's a comfort to have them at hand.

In **Chapter 8: The Renal Diet** of ***What Is It and How Did I Get It? Early Stage Chronic Kidney Disease***, I offer an example of the intricate and annoyingly painstaking little notebook I devised to keep track of my CKD nutrition. Ladies and Gentlemen: I am pleased to announce this is now obsolete!!!

Why not use an app? The one I originally loved and wrote about in ***The Book of Blogs: Moderate Stage Chronic Kidney Disease, Part 2*** was KidneyDiet . Unfortunately, it is no longer available. As I edited ***SlowItDownCKD 2014***, I discovered over 20 other apps.

The theme of today's blog is that life is becoming easier for CKD patients but we've got to keep talking, keep exchanging ideas, keep each other updated about new information. CKD is part of me now, but it sure isn't all of me.

How Sweet It Is... Not

4/28/14   You know those cravings for sweets when you're tired? CKDers get them, too. Once in a very great while, this CKDer gives in to those cravings.

And then I pay for it. My stomach hurts and I need to stay close to what is euphemistically called a restroom in Arizona.

That got me to thinking: what was I doing to my kidneys by giving in to these cravings, even if it were once in a great while? So I researched it, but first I gathered all the information I already had at my fingertips. My starting place? **What Is It and How Did I Get It? Early Stage Chronic Kidney Disease**, of course. It's not just a reference for readers, but for me too.

Bingo! On page 32 {Digital readers, the page numbers will not be helpful to you. Search for the terms, instead.}, I found an explanation of the A1C:

This measures how well your blood sugar has been regulated for the two or three months before the test. That's possible because the glucose adheres to the red blood cells.

So what is glucose and why am I including it in a discussion of sugar and the kidneys, you ask? Turn to page 132 which is part of the *Glossary*. Here, glucose is defined as:

The main sugar found in the blood. In diabetes, the body doesn't adequately control natural and ingested sugar.

Aha! So glucose IS a sugar and it has something to do with diabetes. Diabetes? Back to the A1C. You've heard me be concerned about my A1C for years. That's because below 5.7 is a normal reading. Above 6.5 is diabetes. Anything in-between is pre-diabetes. Guess what my results have been since I've been tested for this. Oh, pre-diabetes, you follow me around like a puppy.

So why should I be so concerned? What was happening to my kidneys?

I do remember reading that too much sugar can damage the lining of your blood vessels. This is something you want to avoid when you're already having problems with your kidneys. The blood vessels carry your blood throughout your body, even if your impaired kidneys have not properly cleaned the blood.

The National Institutes of Health are really good about keeping information reader friendly and allowing the reproduction of their material. This simple explanation of what diabetes can do to your kidneys clarified the issue for me and, hopefully, will do the same for you:

High blood glucose and high blood pressure damage the kidneys' filters. When the kidneys are damaged, proteins leak out of the kidneys into the urine. The urinary albumin test detects this loss of protein in the urine. Damaged kidneys do not do a good job of filtering out wastes and extra fluid. Wastes and fluid build up in your blood instead of leaving the body in urine.

In case you've forgotten what albumin is, see page 129 in the *Glossary* of **What Is It and How Did I Get It? Early Stage Chronic Kidney Disease**.

Albumin: Water soluble protein in the blood.

This blog is turning into an ode to the book rather than a discussion of the effects of too much sugar on the kidneys of a CKDer! I'll stop that right now, folks.

While too much blood glucose can cause the diabetes which may cause Chronic Kidney Disease, the reverse is true, too. CKD can have an effect on your diabetes. If the kidneys are already compromised as far as the part of their job that deals with filtering the blood and now your blood vessel linings are damaged, your body is simply not functioning as it was meant to.

What else can too much sugar do to your body? According to *The Salt* at NPR, it may be affecting your memory more as you age. Agnes Floel of Charite University Medicine in Berlin, the author of a study published in the *New England Journal of Medicine* last year says:

It's possible that blood vessel effects can damage memory. Elevated blood sugar levels damage small and large vessels in the brain, leading to decreased blood and nutrient flow to brain cells….

And then there's sleep apnea. According to a recent EurekAlert! Sleep apnoea has been linked with elevated blood sugar levels, suggesting people with the condition could be at an increased risk of cardiovascular illness and mortality.

The findings of a new study, published online today (3 April 2014) in the *European Respiratory Journal*, add to a growing body of evidence that suggests that sleep apnoea is linked with diabetes.

And heart disease! Let's not forget heart disease! According to Medpage Today

People who had excessive amounts of added sugar in their diet carried greater risks of dying from cardiovascular disease (CVD), researchers found.

This one's for women in my age group.

The most common type of endometrial cancer occurred almost 80% more often in postmenopausal women who regularly consumed sugar-sweetened drinks as compared with women who consumed none, a study found.

This is from another Medpage Today article.

I think I just may have frightened myself enough not to succumb to those sweet cravings. But wait! Carbohydrates also play a part in diabetes. Oh, but that's a blog for another day.

Higher and Higher

5/5/14 "That guideline {e.g. providing a common language for communication among providers, patients and their families, investigators, and policy-makers and a framework for developing a public health approach to affect care and improve outcomes of CKD} led to a paradigm change in the approach to CKD, shifting from an uncommon disease often culminating in kidney failure and treatment by nephrologists to a common condition leading to death from cardiovascular disease. As a result, CKD is now accepted as a worldwide public health problem and the global guideline was developed to address this issue."

This quote is from Andrew S. Levey, MD, co-chair of the NKF KDOQI workgroup that developed the 2002 CKD Guideline and Dr. Gerald J. and Dorothy R. Professor of Medicine at Tufts Medical Center in Boston. You can probably figure out that NKF is the National Kidney Foundation, but you might need a little help with KDOQI. That's the acronym for their Kidney Disease Outcomes Quality Initiative.

2002 was a long time ago, but this statement was issued on December 27th, 2012, which was the night before the release **of Kidney Disease: Improving Global Outcomes (KDIGO).**

By the way, many thanks to the National Kidney Foundation for each time they've asked me to write for them, suggested my name for articles about kidney disease awareness advocates, or offered me suggestions. I've freely quoted from their Kidney.org.

So, CKD is now a common disease. And many people suffering from it die of cardiovascular disease. And hypertension can lead to that... and CKD. Seems pretty circular.

Back to basics. Hypertension or high blood pressure is defined on page 132 of **What Is It and How Did I Get It? Early Stage Chronic Kidney Disease.**

A possible cause of CKD, 140/90 mm Hg is currently considered hypertension, a risk factor for heart disease and stroke, too.

Now, about that 140/90.... According to the National Institutes of Health's National Heart, Lung, and Blood Institute as of January, 2014 If you have diabetes or Chronic Kidney Disease, a blood pressure of 130/80 mmHg or higher is considered HBP.

Not only that, but blood pressure can change depending upon the arm that is being used to measure it, the time of day, whether you've just smoked {Just don't!}, had a cup of coffee or eaten just prior to the test, even if you've just woken up. We all know what worry or stress can do to your blood pressure. It seems even your race can make a difference.

A little less than a year ago, a team at London University College developed a wrist sensor to measure blood pressure as the blood leaves the heart itself. They discovered that blood pressure does not drop as much as thought during the night and that it might be possible to predict heart disease by using this monitoring.

I was particularly interested since I have a wrist monitor that my PCP {primary care physician} prefers I not use, thinking the measurement of the blood passing through the arm arteries more accurate. I'd originally thought this was a wrist monitor but it doesn't measure the blood flowing through the wrist. This was a surprise to me and one I'd like to follow closely.

The Centers for Disease Control and Prevention provides a chart that makes clear why Blacks {or African Americans as they are referred to in the chart} are at 3.5 times the risk of CKD. Look at the numbers, ladies and gents. Hbp {High blood pressure} is the second leading cause of CKD.

Race of Ethnic Group	Men (%)	Women (%)
African Americans	43.0	45.7
Mexican Americans	27.8	28.9
Whites	33.9	31.3
All	34.1	32.7

It's common knowledge that exercise can lower blood pressure, but how many readers know that it can also make your blood pressure medication more effective? On 4/23 of last year, The American Heart Association issued this statement:

Alternative therapies such as aerobic exercise, resistance or strength training and isometric hand grip exercises could help people reduce blood pressure. Biofeedback and device-guided slow breathing reduced blood pressure a small amount. Due to their modest effects, alternative therapies can be used with — not as a replacement for — standard treatment.

Oh, so that's why I didn't give away the isometric hand grips when we gave up 1880s competitive shooting. Good for the trigger finger, just as good for the blood vessels – with proper medication.

Wait a minute. Both the United Kingdom and the United States have populations with almost a third of the people suffering high blood pressure. Think about this. What could this mean?

The Nos(e) Have It

5/12/14 My father had a deviated septum. My daughter has a deviated septum. Why don't I have a deviated septum? Oh right, I'm the lucky one. I only have Chronic Kidney Disease... not that the two are mutually exclusive... or that it's lucky to have CKD.

When it was my father's turn, I was too young to know anything except that my dad was gone overnight. I didn't like that. Now I ask my daughter loads of questions. I don't like that either.

So here I am very ahead of myself and not giving you a clue as to what a deviated septum is. Septum comes from the Latin saeptum, which means

a fence, enclosure, partition

{Thank you, my old academia friend Etymology Online.} We still use that word for the dividing membrane in the nose.

Feel the rigid cartilage under the skin on the outside of your nose. Inside are two chambers separated by the – what else? – septum. Deviated means exactly what you think it does: turned aside. Sometimes you can see the results of a deviated or turned aside septum by looking at a person's nostrils. If one is large and the other very small, it's likely they have a deviated septum.

Sometimes people are born with them, but 80% of the time, they're caused by accidents of one kind or another, or even growing older. Sometimes people don't even know they have a deviated septum. Sometimes it doesn't even matter.

But when you start to experience frequent sinusitis and nosebleeds, it does start to matter. According to The Mayo Clinic:

When a deviated septum is severe, it can block one side of your nose and reduce airflow, causing difficulty breathing. The additional exposure of a deviated septum to the drying effect of airflow through the nose may sometimes contribute to crusting or bleeding in certain individuals.

Some of the symptoms are: preferring to sleep on one side since that allows the larger nostril to get the most air, noisy breathing, the above mentioned nosebleeds and frequent bouts of sinusitis.

Wait, sinusitis? According to Canada.com:

The narrowed nasal passageway caused by a deviated septum can cause mucus to become blocked by preventing the drainage of mucus from a sinus into the nasal cavity. Excess mucus inside the sinuses presents an attractive environment for bacteria, leading to a sinus infection. This in turn causes inflammation of the sinuses (sinusitis), and because it can happen regularly, chronic sinusitis can occur.

Oh, my poor daughter! Frequent nosebleeds, chronic sinusitis, their accompanying post-nasal drip, and headaches. Oh yes, headaches. As I understand it, fluid {can't drain properly due to that deviated septum, remember?} builds up in the sinuses and exerts pressure. Result: headache.

This sounds pretty bad, but there are ways of dealing with a deviated septum. Keep in mind that some people have a mildly deviated septum so they don't do anything for it. Others are troubled by the deviated septum and use medications such as decongestants, nasal sprays, or antihistamines. But when the symptoms are affecting your life and health, surgery is usually suggested.

The following is from MedicineNet.

If a person has a deviated septum and it causes breathing problems or sleep apnea and snoring, surgery may be recommended to repair the septum. Surgery to fix a deviated septum is called a septoplasty, submucous resection of the septum, or septal reconstruction.

Did you notice that this surgery is sometimes necessary so that the sleep apnea – which may be caused by your deviated septum – can be cured?

That's how it affects us as CKD patients. We already have enough problems without sleep apnea! Diabetes, cardiovascular illness, mortality may all be connected to a deviated septum as we know from a recent blog that quoted EurekAlert!

"Sleep apnoea has been linked with elevated blood sugar levels, suggesting people with the condition could be at an increased risk of cardiovascular illness and mortality.

The findings of a new study, published online today (3 April 2014) in the *European Respiratory Journal*, add to a growing body of evidence that suggests that sleep apnoea is linked with diabetes."

Your medical condition is simply not as, well, simple as you think with CKD. Deviated septum may lead to sleep apnea, which may lead to diabetes, or any of the other outcomes listed above.

Okay, we're ready to take a look at the surgery now. I found this at Deviated Septum.org via a simple Yahoo search:

Septoplasty is the surgical treatment which is preferred by doctors worldwide to correct a deviated septum. The surgery is done entirely through the nostrils, thus no external bruising occurs. During the surgery the portion of the septum which are [sic] extremely deviated will be re-adjusted or realigned or removed completely.

Sometimes people do have a nose job {rhinoplasty} at the same time. This completely changes the shape of the nose. But let's not judge here; maybe the adjustments made to the deviated septum would make the appearance of the finished product unacceptable to the patient.

A Foggy Day... in Your Brain

5/19/14 I don't know about you, but I thoroughly enjoy my 16 ounces of coffee a day. I savor it and draw those two cups out as long as I can. I relish the taste and adore the aroma. And, I thought they would cut through what I've discovered is called 'brain fog.'

I receive daily notices of who posted what where on the Facebook CKD support groups. I noticed a question about brain fog and was surprised at the responses. The question asked who else suffered this cloudiness of thought and what stage they were in.

Once I understood what brain fog was, I imagined the responses would all mention end stage. They didn't. I saw all stages from 2 through 5 mentioned. I was grabbed by the fact that no one in stage 1 had responded and that's when brain fog became the topic of today's blog. According to integrative medicine expert Dr. Isaac Eliaz, when experiencing brain fog:

...people feel as if there is a thick fog dampening their mind. While the medical and mental health establishments don't generally recognize brain fog as a condition, it's a surprisingly common affliction that affects people of all ages. Symptoms include pervasive absentmindedness, muddled thought processes, poor memory recall, difficulty processing information, disorientation, fatigue, and others.

While this is interesting, what does it have to do with renal disease? I know there are readers who only want to read about subjects that affect us as sufferers of this disease. I know because I get a good laugh when they ask what a particular blog has to do with renal disease. That's why I write the blog.

So I did what I love to do: researched the topic. Here's what I found at naturopathconnect.com which offered me my first insight into how our kidneys and brain fog are connected.

Make sure your liver and kidneys are not overloaded or congested. When your liver and kidneys are not functioning well, they are less able to clear your system of the multitude of toxins that float around in your bloodstream. When your body is overloaded with toxins, your brain suffers as well....Dehydration may be a key factor in less-than-optimal kidney function, so water is essential to keep the kidneys in tip-top shape.

Got it – toxins. Uh, what toxins? And how do they affect the brain, I wondered. Back to researching.

Dr. Martin Morrell of healthtap.com offered an explanation. However, this is not an endorsement of him or the site. I am not a fan of asking online doctors unfamiliar with your particular medical history for advice.

... if your blood urea increases, which is supposed to be cleared by your kidneys, this 'poison' will affect the ability of the brain to work properly.

Oh, blood urea. Well that explains it. But how can I explain blood urea? I'll allow the experts to do that. The UK site Patient has the simplest explanation:

Urea is a waste product formed from the breakdown of proteins. Urea is usually passed out in the urine. A high blood level of urea ('uraemia') indicates that the kidneys may not be working properly, or that you are dehydrated (have a low body water content).

In the U.S., we call this test B.U.N. or Blood Urea Nitrogen Test. So as I understand it, if your protein intake is high, more urea is produced. But since your kidneys are already compromised by CKD, the toxins remaining in your body are not eliminated as well and are still in the blood that flows through your brain. That's logical.

The more urea remaining in your system, the more sluggish your brain. It does sound like a perfectly formed 'if-then' equation from probability theory. The only difference here is that this is not a theory, but, rather, what we may encounter as CKD patients.

What to do? What to do? Obviously, keeping our protein intake low will help. My renal diet limits me to five ounces of protein a day. I rarely ingest more protein than that. Well, bully for me! So how else can I alleviate my sometimes brain fog?

I was all over the web on this one and found that besides what I was already doing for my CKD, I could also avoid heavy metal {and I always thought that was a kind of music} exposure, use a blue light, get myself some natural sun light, check my medication side effects and lots more. This is the stuff of several blogs.

It's real. Brain fog could be affecting you, especially if you have CKD. And from what I've read, once you've gotten your CKD slowed down as much as possible, the other 'fixes' are easy.

From The Military to Potatoes

5/26/14 Some of our present protectors have CKD. This is how I discovered that fact:

The National Institutes of Health offered a particular Funding Opportunity Application [FOA] on December 1st, 2011, with the first submission being accepted on January 14, 2012.

The goal of this FOA is to encourage Research Project Grant (R01) applications on prevention and treatment of obesity, diabetes, and Chronic Kidney Disease in military personnel (active duty and retired) and their families.

Notice "active duty" in that sentence. Both The National Institute of Diabetes and Digestive and Kidney Diseases (NIDDK) and the Eunice Kennedy Shriver National Institute of Child Health and Human Development (NICHD) participate in this study. Unfortunately, my attempts to follow up on the study consistently brought me back to the FOA.

The Department of Defense's Instruction for Medical Standards for Appointment, Enlistment, or Induction in the Military Services …Establishes medical standards, which, if not met, are grounds for rejection for military service. Other standards may be prescribed for a mobilization for a national emergency….

As of September 13, 2011, according to Change 1 of this Instruction, the following was included.

Current or history of acute (580) nephritis or chronic (582) Chronic Kidney Disease of any type.

Until this date, Chronic Kidney Disease was not mentioned. I cannot explain the seeming contradiction between the FOA and the Directive.

Although, when my daughter Nima – researcher par excellence – asked me if I had a particular request for Mother's Day, I asked her for research on the early history of CKD. She found there wasn't very much until fairly recently. The fact that the first set of clinical practice guidelines (K/DOQI comprised *Chronic Kidney Disease: Evaluation, Classification and Stratification*) wasn't published until February, 2002, may account for the lack of information from the military.

While my information is inconclusive {at best}, I sincerely hope that our warriors – whether on active duty or retired – have the same kind of care for their CKD as those of us who are civilians do. Thank you again… and again…and again to our protectors, including my Bear.

Someone we're close with invited us to brunch. When my eyes lit up at the sight of baby potatoes {I'm Russian by heritage.}, he commented, "I leached the potatoes, sort of."

Let's go back to basics here for a moment. On page 134 {Do a word search instead of relying on the page number if you own a digital copy of the book.} of **What Is It and How Did I Get It? Early Stage Chronic Kidney Disease**, I define potassium as

One of the electrolytes, important because it counteracts sodium's effect on blood pressure.

Dictionary.com tells us that electrolytes are

…any of certain inorganic compounds, mainly sodium, potassium, magnesium, calcium, chloride, and bicarbonate, that dissociate in biological fluids into ions capable of conducting electrical currents and constituting a major force in controlling fluid balance within the body. Potassium is necessary for the nerves and muscles. The heart is a muscle. But our compromised kidneys cannot eliminate enough potassium from the blood before it travels back to the heart. This may lead to heart attack… or kidney failure. It's a chicken and the egg kind of thing.

These are the acceptable values of potassium in your blood. As you can see, there is a difference in the values for adults and children of various ages. The chart is from Everyday Health.

Potassium (K)

Adults:	3.5-5.2 milliequivalents per liter (mEq/L) or 3.5-5.2 millimoles per liter (mmol/L)
Children:	3.4-4.7 mEq/L or 3.4-4.7 mmol/L
Infants:	4.1-5.3 mEq/L or 4.1-5.3 mmol/L
Newborns:	3.7-5.9 mEq/L or 3.7-5.9 mmol/L

I went to Kidneys.com to see what, if any, the symptoms of high potassium levels are:

- Nausea
- Weakness
- Numbness or tingling
- Slow pulse
- Irregular heartbeat
- Heart failure

Now, keep in mind that at early stages of CKD you may not have high levels of potassium. The idea is to keep your levels low so that you do not do damage to yourself since your kidneys are not doing such a great of eliminating it.

But here's the kicker: raising potassium levels could lower your blood pressure. Remember high blood pressure is the second leading cause of CKD. Just like riding a bicycle, it's all a matter of balance.

Since being diagnosed, I've leached the potassium out of potatoes by cutting them into pieces, soaking them in water for four hours, changing the water, and letting them soak again or soaking them in the refrigerator overnight. That's a lot of time involvement, time I knew my almost son-in-law did not have in his schedule.

So I researched for a less time consuming method that I could mention to him. I wanted to eat what he prepared, but only if it didn't cause my CKD to progress. I was surprised to discover that the only effective way to leach potatoes and other vegetables is to double boil them. Thank you to Kidneycoach for this new, researched, effective method.

However, I find that new research disparaging. Sure, the potassium is out, but boiled potatoes? And other vegetables since all contain some level of potassium? How is that appetizing? Then again, I like being alive, I like not being on dialysis, so I will just cope.

Your Thyroid and Chronic Kidney Disease Have Something Going On

6/2/14 Today's blog was written at the request of a reader. The deal is I write a blog about hyperthyroid and its connection to Chronic Kidney Disease and she goes directly to her nephrologist to ask him the same questions she asked me.

While I'm a good researcher, I am not a doctor and that's who should be asked your CKD questions. Come to think of it, any time you receive any well-meant advice about this disease, check with your nephrologist first… even if you admire the brain of the person giving the advice. Let's do our usual go-back-to-basics-first. The thyroid, according to WebMD,

… secretes several hormones, collectively called thyroid hormones. The main hormone is thyroxine, also called T4. Thyroid hormones act throughout the body, influencing metabolism, growth and development, and body temperature. During infancy and childhood, adequate thyroid hormone is crucial for brain development.

There doesn't seem to be anything alarming there, so let's go to the T4. I turned to **_What Is It and How Did I Get It? Early Stage Chronic Kidney Disease_** for information about this and found it on page 23 {Usual reminder: digital book owners, use a word search rather than a page}.

What this test is really for is to see if the T3 test comes back abnormal. If it does, the lab needs to run another thyroid test. That test, the T4, is a further thyroid test which looks for specific causes of the abnormality.

Ah, so we need to be tested via a blood draw to see if there is an abnormality in our thyroid function. Without getting technical, the abnormalities could be hypothyroid or hyperthyroid. As a former English teacher, I know hypo is a prefix {a group of letters added to the beginning of a word that changes its definition} that means under, while hyper means over.

My reader's question was about hyperthyroid, but for the sake of completeness, I'll include the symptoms of hypothyroid.

1. Cold hands and feet
2. Chronic fatigue
3. Lethargy and fatigue
4. Emotional instability
5. Depression

Hyperthyroid is not as common as hypothyroid and presents different symptoms.

1. Sweating
2. Anxiety and Excitability
3. Thirst
4. Racing heart
5. Hunger
6. Muscle weakness
7. Shortness of breath
8. High blood pressure
9. Insomnia
10. Weight loss

Numbers 7 & 8 caught my eye immediately since they seem to have something to do with CKD.

The diagnose I was specifically asked about is hyperthyroid, renal. We already know renal means kidney, so this deals with how the overactive thyroid affects the kidneys. Remember that hormones travel through the blood and that the thyroid produces a hormone. Too much of that hormone produces the above symptoms.

As I understand it {And, again, I am not a doctor} – as mentioned – the thyroid produces a hormone which is released into the blood, while the kidneys filter the blood. If you have CKD, your kidneys are not functioning as well as they should. If you have hyperthyroid, you are producing extra thyroid hormone that your compromised kidneys cannot purge from your blood as well as they should.

The following quote from Wellness Resources encapsulates the interplay between the kidneys and the thyroid.

A considerable body of science now links thyroid problems and kidney problems in a "chicken and egg" manner.

So yes, the CKD could have caused the hyperthyroid, renal, and vice versa. However, hypothyroid does seem to be more common than hyperthyroid.

Baby, It's Hot Outside

6/9/14 I just caught up to the fact that it's June. No, it wasn't the calendar that told me, but the temperature. We live in Arizona and its hot, dry heat or not. That means cooling off any way you can. I was offered some filtered water. Did I want ice? I was asked.

I immediately shook my head. "CKD, no ice, please."

My former colleague asked me why and I immediately knew what I was going to blog about today.

For years, I've misunderstood something my nephrologist said. I heard, "Don't use ice." What he really said was something like, "If you use ice, you need to count the cubes in your fluid intake."

I've spent time since Saturday researching the ice question and found nothing about avoiding ice. I did find one warning about cold beverages from DaVita:

Be careful of very cold beverages, which can cause stomach cramps. The lesson I learned from this misunderstanding of what I thought I heard is to recheck what you think you know every once in a while. After all, I thought I had the diet down pat.

Hah! I forgot that I was terrified when I was first diagnosed and thinking I was going to die imminently. I adhered strictly to what I heard and, apparently, adhered just as strictly to what I thought I'd heard.

Wait a minute… maybe I need not have avoided the heat, either. I researched that, too. Just as with ice, I found a general warning about the elderly, but nothing specific to CKD.

"With the elderly, the heat accumulates in their bodies over hours to days. If you have a long heat spell, the elderly person accumulates heat through each of those days because they can't really eliminate or dissipate the heat," explains Dr. Crocker. "Sometimes it's because of a medication, sometimes it's a lack of mobility, or in some cases the older you get, the less active your sweat glands are, so it becomes harder and harder for you to eliminate heat."

This is from The Austin Diagnostic Clinic.

But, again, there was nothing specific to CKDers in the quote above. In thinking about it, I began to wonder if the risk of dehydration from the summer heat is the problem for us.

According to The National Kidney Fund:

Kidneys can become damaged if they are not getting good blood flow. This can happen if you become dehydrated or seriously ill.

Aha! This was starting to make sense. WebMD explains this for us:

Usually your body can reabsorb fluid from your blood and other body tissues. But by the time you become severely dehydrated, you no longer have enough fluid in your body to get blood to your organs, and you may go into shock, which is a life-threatening condition.

Okay, so we know we need to drink fluids, especially in hot weather. Our kidneys are already having a hard time cleaning our blood effectively and we are reabsorbing ineffectively cleaned blood prior to this point of dehydration.

But how do we know if we're becoming dehydrated? What are the symptoms? I turned to my standby, The Mayo Clinic for the symptoms of mild dehydration.

- Dry, sticky mouth
- Sleepiness or tiredness — children are likely to be less active than usual
- Thirst
- Decreased urine output
- No wet diapers for three hours for infants
- Few or no tears when crying
- Dry skin
- Headache
- Constipation
- Dizziness or lightheadedness

And then I laughed. I experience one or more of those symptoms at one time or another. The clinic does make the extremely helpful point that the color of your urine is a good indicator of dehydration. If it's clear or light in color, you're fine. If it's dark, start drinking! Interestingly enough, having CKD is already a risk factor for dehydration so let's not make it worse for ourselves.

So how do we prevent dehydration? What can we do if we can see it starting?

Obviously, drinking more fluids will help. I'm limited to 64 ounces in a day, but I get creative in summer. Sometimes, I will have that half cup of ice cream. Watermelon magically appears on the table. Now that I realize I don't have to avoid ice, it too will become part of the anti-dehydration campaign in our house.

I'm not sure if this is common knowledge, but dehydration can also cause kidney stones. If you don't have the fluid in your body to prevent crystallization, crystallization is more apt to happen. Kidney stones are Stones caused in the urinary tract and kidney when crystals adhere to each other. Most of those in the kidneys are made of calcium.

That's from ***What Is It and How Did I Get It? Early Stage Chronic Kidney Disease***, p. 133.

Their Father's Food

6/16/14 Bear chose the menu for Father's Day and it included many non-renal diet foods.

Thank you Wedliny Domowe for this information:

Ham is a processed meat. It can be cured in a number of ways, but most include the use of salt, and nitrites, which themselves are either sodium or potassium. The dry method of curing uses salt, while the wet method uses brine. And what is brine but a solution of sodium in water? And then there's smoking. {Ack! Smoke contains formaldehyde and alcohol.} We know as CKDers that we need to limit our sodium intake. As I wrote in ***What Is It and How Did I Get It? Early Stage Chronic Kidney Disease,*** pages 73-4

Basically, sodium balances fluid levels outside your cells. You need it because it is responsible for watering your cells. This watering is the prompt for potassium to dump waste [cell process by-products] from your cells....If you have damaged kidneys and cannot excrete most of the sodium you ingest, you're up against higher blood pressure which may worsen your CKD which may further cut down on your elimination of sodium and so on and so forth in an ever spiraling cycle. In addition, for CKD patients, too much sodium causes fluid retention, thereby causing swelling, further resulting in weight gain, leading to shortness of breath.

And let's not forget that high blood pressure is the second leading cause of Chronic Kidney Disease.

Well, what about the potassium in the nitrite used in preserving the ham? Why do CKDers have to limit the amount of potassium they ingest? By the way, too much sodium can increase your need for potassium.

But isn't potassium good for you? After all, it does help the heart, muscles, and our beloved kidneys function normally as well as dumping wastes from our cells. Here's the kicker, an excess of potassium can cause irregular heartbeat and even heart attack.

We are not your everyday people whose kidneys can filter any excess potassium from our bodies. We have compromised kidney function which could mean a buildup in potassium. No wonder CKD may lead to cardiovascular problems!

I'm almost afraid to look at the rest of Bear's Father's Day menu. He also requested cold cuts of roast beef. Uh-oh, that's another cured meat. Cold cuts also tend to be fattier cuts and have nitrates, which are different than the nitrites discussed above.

According to Dictionary.com:

a nitrate is a salt or ester {That's an organic compound.} of nitric acid.

Wait a minute! Nitric acid is a corrosive liquid, as most of us learned way back in high school.

And, as Dr. Veeraish Chauhan {one of the nephrologists in Florida that received a donation of the book this past March when I was there} wrote in his April 6, 2013 blog

... red meat could be a big source of uric acid, which has been shown to be associated with worsening of CKD.

Red meat contains cholesterol. Fattier cuts contain more cholesterol. This substance can clog the arteries, leading to heart problems. We already have a higher risk of heart problems simply because we have CKD. Why raise the risk???

And then we have the sweet potato casserole. Sweet potatoes? I don't remember the last time I had one of those. Talk about potassium overload! We already discussed the CKDers' problems with that.

Well, what about the green bean casserole? I didn't have to eat the crispy, fried onions on top of it. But it's in creamed mushroom soup. Oh, right. Creamed soup is high in phosphorous, as The National Kidney Foundation tells us, although phosphorus is necessary to work with calcium for healthy bones.

High phosphorus levels can cause damage to your body. Extra phosphorus causes body changes that pull calcium out of your bones, making them weak. High phosphorus and calcium levels also lead to dangerous calcium deposits in blood vessels, lungs, eyes, and heart. Phosphorus and calcium control is very important for your overall health.

The orange mimosas seemed to delight everyone but Abby. I didn't even try one. I.just.don't.drink. Too much alcoholism in my family history. Anyway, while the orange juice in this drink didn't seem to be a problem, the champagne was actually good for us, according to the National Institutes of Health.

Their MedlinePlus posted new findings about the benefits of wine. Champagne is a wine. Surprise! If you have CKD, wine in moderation may help protect you from that heart disease you've at risk of.

I am not even going to analyze the carrot cake from Cheesecake Factory. That is so bad for you on so many levels! I am so glad I researched these foods AFTER the celebratory meal so I wasn't tempted to spout this information to those enjoying the food.

Not ON the Water, IN It

6/23/14   It's hot, 112 degrees already and summer has just started. Much as I'd love to, I can't stay in the house writing all day, every day. I also need to exercise on a daily basis... as do you if you have Chronic Kidney Disease.

What's that? Why do you have to exercise if you have CKD, you ask? Let's go back to **What Is It and How Did I Get It? Early Stage Chronic Kidney Disease**, page 100, for the answer to that one. {Digital book owners, don't forget to use the search document function instead of the page number.}

I knew exercise was important to control my weight. It would also improve my blood pressure and lower my cholesterol and triglyceride levels. The greater your triglycerides, the greater the risk of increasing your creatinine. There were other benefits, too, although you didn't have to have CKD to enjoy them: better sleep, and improved muscle function and strength. But, as with everything else you do that might impinge upon your health, check with your doctor before you start exercising.

I researched, researched and researched again. Each explanation of what exercise does for the body was more complicated than the last one I read. Keeping it simple, basically, there's a compound released by voluntary muscle contraction. It tells the body to repair itself and grow stronger. The idea is to start exercising slowly and then intensify your activity.

I've mentioned water walking as an exercise and gotten quite a few questions about it. I have to admit I'd never heard of it before I moved to Arizona and met Bear. His house is in a senior citizen community that has a community center with a water walking pool.

It was exciting to be doing something I'd never done before and I questioned him unmercifully, although he kept telling me you get in a pool that has lanes and walk. I could not visualize it, so I went online to see what it looked like. Then I couldn't imagine what it would feel like, especially for someone who always wants to be near water rather than in it.

The pool was enormous to my water walking pool virgin eyes. There were shady parts and sunny parts. Uh-oh, I was going to have to get a hat with a bigger brim to protect my neck and shoulders from the sun, too. Oh, and water soluble sunscreen.

I couldn't make sense of the arrows on the pool floor and the curvy shoulder high dividing walls between lanes until I was actually in the pool. I started out in waist high water following the arrows and keeping in the lanes they pointed to on different sides of the dividers until I found myself in chin high water when we completed our first circuit. Now it all made sense. It was just like traffic lanes and directional markings on the road when you drive! Of course, waist and chin high are relative. I'm 5'5', so Bear's 5'10" meant the water was not as high on him.

There's another benefit to water walking if you have arthritis. You've read my complaints about arthritis here and even in the *Wall Street Journal* column by Laura Landro about CKD Awareness activists {I still prefer being called an advocate}. If you missed it, you can read that article in their archives. It was printed on January 12th, 2014.

I went to the site of The Arthritis Foundation and read the following.

Like all water exercises, water walking is easy on the joints. "The water's buoyancy supports the body's weight, which reduces stress on the joints and minimizes pain," says Jones {an aquatic coordinator}. "And it's still a great workout. Water provides 12 times the resistance of air, so as you walk, you're really strengthening and building muscle." You do not bear weight while swimming and walking, however, so you'll still need to add some bone-building workouts to your routine.

My almost constantly complaining knees were quiet in the water walking pool. My slightly painful hip didn't seem to hurt. And, best of all, my elbows weren't aching. I'm sold. What makes it even better is that water walking strengthens your muscles.

The bottom of the pool is purposely rough to prevent slips. After one circuit without water shoes, I knew I'd have to get some. While they were not severely damaged, I did notice annoying little scrapes and cuts on the soles of my feet, especially my toes.

That probably means I was walking on my toes, something The Mayo Clinic suggests you NOT do.

In water that's about waist-high, walk across the pool swinging your arms like you do when walking on land. Avoid walking on your tiptoes, and keep your back straight. Tighten your abdominal muscles to avoid leaning too far forward or to the side.

I'll also have to work on tightening my abdominals since I walked into the wall or the dividers a few times. I knew I wasn't drunk {I don't drink.}, so now I know why this happened.

A non-medical site, Ask.com, had some information about how you can water walk in any water. After all, not everyone has access to a water walking pool.

• Walk forward and backward with short steps, long steps, average steps, or step kicks.
• Move in a pattern of a circle or square. Be sure to go in both directions to balance the demands on your body.

Life Is Just a Bowl of Cherries

6/30/14   Here I was all ready to write about sulfur drugs and CKD or hearing and CKD when I received an email from a loyal reader who'd just bought some good looking Bing cherries but wasn't sure whether to eat them or not. We all know that cherries simply don't last that long, so this one's for her.

The big issue about eating cherries when you have Chronic Kidney Disease is their potassium content. I went straight to **What Is It and How Did I Get It? Early Stage Chronic Kidney Disease** to see what I'd written about this. In the *Glossary* {on page 134} I found this definition.

One of the electrolytes, important because it counteracts sodium's effect on blood pressure.

While that's true, we're going to need more to help the reader out. So I turned to *Chapter 8: The Renal Diet* {page 75}.

Potassium is something you need to limit when you have CKD despite the fact that potassium not only dumps waste from your cells but also helps the kidneys, heart and muscles to function normally. Too much potassium can cause irregular heartbeat and even heart attack. This can be the most immediate danger of not limiting your potassium….
…Check your blood tests. 3.5-5 is considered a safe level of potassium. You may have a problem if your blood level of potassium is 5.1-6 and you definitely need to attend to it if it's above 6. Speak to your nephrologist ….

I checked with the National Kidney Foundation about those levels just to be sure they hadn't changed since the book was published. They haven't.

That got me to wondering why cherries are considered good for the general population, but not CKD patients. So, of course, I did a little research. Green and Healthy suggests those without kidney disease eat cherries for the following reason.

According to research from Michigan State University tart cherries contain anthocyanins {thought you might like to know this means natural pain relieving and anti-inflammatory properties}, bioflavonoids, which inhibit the enzymes Cyclooxygenase-1 and -2, and prevent inflammation in the body. These compounds have similar activity as aspirin, naproxen and ibuprofen.

Sounds good to me since we can't take some of those pain relievers, but cherries have the same effect. Something was nagging at me though. Back to **What Is It and How Did I Get It? Early Stage Chronic Kidney Disease**. As I read page 3, I realized why.

The problem with unregulated minerals, such as sodium and potassium is that these minerals are needed to remain healthy but too much in the bloodstream becomes toxic. The kidneys remove these toxins and change them into urine that enters the bladder via the ureter.

Well, healthy kidneys do, but just how effective are your compromised kidneys at doing this job? I went to DaVita, but in addition to the usual warnings about potassium levels, I found the following.

- 1/2 cup serving fresh sweet cherries = 0 mg sodium, 160 mg potassium, 15 mg phosphorus
- Cherries have been shown to reduce inflammation when eaten daily. They are also packed with antioxidants and phytochemicals that protect the heart.

Does that mean they're good for CKD patients?

From my reading, I've also garnered the information that cherries can help with iron deficiencies, lower blood pressure, improve sleep, help with gout, and lower the risk of heart disease.

Or can they? Remember that too much potassium can actually cause an irregular heartbeat or possibly stop your heart.

For the reader who asked and all the rest of us, I'm sure I've only added to your confusion. Watch your potassium levels. Look them up on your last blood test. Why not give your nephrologist a call, too, just to be sure. Do you have a renal nutritionist? He or she would know far better than I since this question of whether to eat the cherries or not is so individualized.

Then we have stages. I am stage 3, which I used to think was early stage {Hence, my first book's title.} but now realize is moderate stage. I don't know what stage our questioner is, but I do know the dietary rules change when you reach end stage and I'm going to guess they're even different for those on different kinds of dialysis and those who are transplants.

So this reader's question is sort of asking me which sexual position is best for her. I'm purposely being provocative here so that you'll see just how individualized the renal diet is. What's best for you depends on your needs. Call the nutritionist!

Knowing End Stage Renal Disease is not my area of expertise, I took a peek at National Kidney and Urologic Diseases Information Clearinghouse (NKUDIC), A service of the National Institute of Diabetes and Digestive and Kidney Diseases (NIDDK), National Institutes of Health (NIH) anyway to see what dialysis patients can eat. Apparently, potassium could be a problem here, too. This is what I found:

Potassium is a mineral found in many foods, especially milk, fruits, and vegetables. It affects how steadily your heart beats. Healthy kidneys keep the right amount of potassium in the blood to keep the heart beating at a steady pace. Potassium levels can rise between dialysis sessions and affect your heartbeat. Eating too much potassium can be very dangerous to your heart. It may even cause death.

Okay, cherries can be a problem. Then I started wondering if it mattered what type of cherries they were. I found at least 18 different kinds, but none of the websites discussed potassium.

I learned more about cherries and potassium than I thought I wanted to. I'm sure you did, too, but I offer you the same advice I offered the loyal reader with the question: check with your renal nutritionist or nephrologist – always. I am not a doctor, but rather someone who researches CKD on a layman's level. Loyal reader, thanks for asking.

I Can Hear the Blood Rushing in My Ears

7/7/14   Hope you had a wonderful Independence Day weekend. During ours, my blog was in the back of my mind. It's always in the back of my mind. Which is why I can't stop writing it, by the way. This weekend, I kept thinking about the subtle connection between hearing and Chronic Kidney Disease.

The topic came about in the usual way: I complained of hearing poorly and my ever vigilant primary care doctor suggested I might want to have my hearing tested by an audiologist. This was right after I passed the Medicare Annual Wellness Visit hearing test with flying colors despite my complaints.

Off I went to take a hearing test for the third time in five years. Her assessment was that my hearing was just fine. Go figure, but she did applaud me for telling her I had CKD {and sleep apnea, but that's another story…uh, blog}.

Why did I do that you ask? Well, as I wrote on my March 15th, 2011, blog during National Kidney Month:

Research shows that hearing loss is common in people with moderate Chronic Kidney Disease. As published in the American Journal of Kidney Diseases and highlighted on the National Kidney Foundation web site, a team of Australian researchers found that older adults with moderate Chronic Kidney Disease (CKD) have a higher prevalence of hearing loss than those of the same age without CKD.

How moderate CKD and hearing are connected is another matter, one that apparently isn't as well documented. Here's what I found at Hear It.org which has an online hearing test – and not most, but all of the other sites I searched. This comes from the same study I used in my 2011 blog. That study was completed in 2010… four years ago. University of Sydney said:

The link between hearing loss and CKD can be explained by structural and functional similarities between tissues in the inner ear and in the kidney. Additionally, toxins that accumulate in kidney failure can damage nerves, including those in the inner ear. Another reason for this connection is that kidney disease and hearing loss share common risk factors, including diabetes, high blood pressure and advanced age.

Suddenly it became clear. If toxins are – well – toxic to our bodies, that includes our ears. My old friend The Online Etymology Dictionary tells us the word toxic is derived directly from Late Latin toxicus, which means "poisoned."

Now I got it. Moderate CKD could be poisoning our bodies with a buildup of toxins. Our ears and the nerves in them are part of our body. Damaged nerves may cause hearing loss. I'd just never thought of it that way before. Sometimes all it takes is that one last piece of the puzzle to fall in place.

Hmmm. High blood pressure is the second most common leading cause of CKD and it can also lead to hearing loss. Let's take a look at that. According to WebMD

Certain illnesses, such as heart disease, high blood pressure, and diabetes, put ears at risk by interfering with the ears' blood supply. I went right to **What Is It and How Did I Get It? Early Stage Chronic Kidney Disease** to figure out how. On page 97 {You know the drill: digital readers use the search function.}, there is a diagram from The National Institute of Diabetes and Digestive and Kidney Diseases, National Institutes of Health that demonstrates how high blood pressure is caused... and if you read on, you'll read about the problems high blood pressure causes.

This is the sentence that clarified the issue for me {page 99}.

Humans have 10 pints of blood that are pumped by the heart through the arteries to all the other parts of the bodies.

That would include the ears. Moderate CKD might mean that blood is tainted by the toxins our compromised kidneys could not rid us of.

I had been hoping for more recent research, but sometimes you just have to deal with what you get.

How I Connect Coyotes and CKD

7/14/14   When Bear was helping me unload the groceries from my car last night, he pointed out a coyote casually walking down the street. We're only a quarter of a mile from an arroyo {same thing as a wash, a gulley that seasonally fills up with rushing rain water} and often see wild life there, but other than bunnies and Gambrel Quail, not in front of the house.

This means Bella needs to stay in the house from before dusk until after dawn since those are prime hunting times for the coyote. Her dog door was closed last night. While she is a medium sized dog, I wouldn't be surprised if a pack of coyotes could devour her... and that's why they're on our block.

These creatures are hungry and they want red meat. They're adaptable and will eat anything when they're hungry enough – even garbage – but 90% of their diet consists of red meat when they can find it. Notice I'm not citing any websites here. This is common knowledge when you live in the desert, something I've done for the last dozen years.

The coyote sighting got me to thinking. They eat red meat. Humans do, too. Yet, as Chronic Kidney Disease patients we're urged away from this practice. I accept it, but I've forgotten why and thought you might have, too.

As usual, let's start at the beginning. Precisely what is 'red meat'? According to the Bing Dictionary, red meat is,

meat that is red when raw: meat that is relatively dark red in color when raw, e.g. beef or lamb.

I don't eat lamb and never have due to some childhood questioning as to why a child should eat another child. Red meat was the staple of the family's diet when I grew up and no meal was considered complete without it. That's not the case now.

WebMD has a truly illuminating three page article debating the merits and demerits of red meat. Most of it deals with the protein and fat content. That is something that should concern us as CKD patients. {It also explains why pork is considered a red meat rather than a white meat as a former colleague tried to convince me.}

Okay, so fat – and hence, cholesterol – is something that could adversely affect your heart, not great for anyone including us. But, as CKD sufferers, it's more the protein content of red meat that concerns us right now.

In **What Is It and How Did I Get It? Early Stage Chronic Kidney Disease,** protein is defined as:

Amino acids arranged in chains joined by peptide bonds to form a compound, important because some proteins are hormones, enzymes, and antibodies.

 That's on pages 134-5 for those of you with a print copy of the book. Those of you with a digital copy, use the word search function.
That definition says a lot. Let's take it bit by bit. Amino acids, simply put, are:

any one of many acids that occur naturally in living things and that include some which form proteins.

Thank you, Merriam Webster Dictionary. Did you notice that they may form proteins? Keep that in mind.

So what are peptide bonds, then? This is a bit more complicated, so I went to Education Portal for the most easily understood definition:

Peptide bonds are the key linkages found in proteins. These bonds connect amino acids and provide one of the key foundations for protein structure.

Again, proteins. This is a bit circular, but the important point here is that both are involved in the production of protein.

The renal diet I follow restricts my daily protein intake to five ounces a day, but why? Back to **What Is It and How Did I Get It? Early Stage Chronic Kidney Disease,** page77 this time.

So, why is protein limited? One reason is that it is the source of a great deal of phosphorus. Another is that a number of nephrons were already destroyed before you were even diagnosed. Logically, those that remain compensate for those that are no longer viable. The remaining nephrons are doing more work than they were meant to. Just like a car that is pushed too hard, there will be constant deterioration if you don't stop pushing. The idea is to stop pushing your remaining nephrons to work even harder in an attempt to slow down the advancement of your CKD. Restricting protein is a way to reduce the nephrons' work.

Your kidneys have about a million nephrons, which are those tiny structures that produce urine as part of the body's waste removal process. Each of them has a glomerulus or network of capillaries. This is where the blood from the renal artery is filtered. The glomerulus is connected to a renal tubule, something so small that it is microscopic. The renal tubule is attached to a collection area. The blood is filtered. Then the waste goes through the tubules to have water and chemicals balanced according to the body's present needs. Finally, the waste is voided via your urine to the tune of 50 gallons of fluid filtered by the kidneys DAILY. The renal vein uses blood vessels to take most of the blood back into the body.

For those of you who may have forgotten, phosphorus isn't troublesome in early or moderate stage CKD, but can be in Stages 4 and 5.

Phosphorus works in conjunction with calcium to keep our bones and teeth healthy, but it has other jobs, too. Compromised kidneys cannot filter out enough of this, though. That can lead to calcification in parts of the body.

It's the Long Promised Sulfa Blog!

7/21/14 Since I mentioned sulfa drugs in a blog a few weeks ago, I've been asked some questions, including one wanting to know if these drugs could have caused a particular reader's CKD. Although I used the British spelling, I also wrote about my experience with sulfa drugs in ***What Is It and How Did I Get It? Early Stage Chronic Kidney Disease*** {page 90}:

I knew I wasn't feeling well at all, so I called my primary care physician for an appointment. Her medical assistant [M.A.] told me my doctor was out of town for a week and to go to the urgent care center near my home since, as a CKD patient, I should not wait. When I told the receptionist at the urgent care center that I had CKD, she sent me to the emergency room at the local hospital in case I needed blood tests or scans for which the urgent care center was unequipped. The hospital did run a scan and blood tests. This way, they were able to see if I had an infection, blockage or some imbalance that might not only make me feel sick but worsen the CKD.

I already knew I had a higher than usual white blood cell count from my previous fasting blood test for the nephrologist about a month before the emergency room visit. He'd felt it was not significantly high enough to indicate an infection but was, rather, a function of a woman's anatomy. Women have shorter internal access to the bladder, as opposed to those of men. Looked like my nephrologist might have misjudged.

However, he quickly picked up that the medication prescribed by the emergency room physicians, despite my having reiterated several times that I have CKD, was a sulfur based drug. He quickly made a sub-stitution, saving possible further damage to my kidneys. The hospital insisted I only had Stage 2, so this was a safe drug for me. I was nervous about this as soon as they became defensive about prescribing this medication. You need to stick to your guns about being taken seriously when it comes to CKD.

All right, let's go back to basics, first. The Medical Dictionary defines sulfa drug as:

Any sulfa-based antibiotic, in particular sulfonamides

Great. Now we just need to know what sulfonamides are. The same dictionary tells us these are:

medicines that prevent the growth of bacteria in the body
and that they are frequently used with urinary tract infections. Yet, there's also a warning that people with kidney disease should be sure to warn their doctors about their kidney disease should one of these drugs be prescribed.

Well, why do you need to avoid such medications with CKD? As you already know, compromised kidneys don't do the job they were meant to do as well as they did before we had CKD when it comes to eliminating drugs from our bodies. The kidneys are the organs that clear this particular drug from the body, not the liver {which is another organ that can clear drugs from your body}. That means the drug may build up… and cause problems.

Here's one of those problems from MedicineNet:

Other rare side effects include liver damage, low white blood cell count (leucopenia), low platelet count (thrombocytopenia), and anemia. Formation of urinary crystals which may damage the kidney and may cause blood in the urine. Adequate hydration is needed to prevent the formation of urinary crystals.

We are already prone to anemia since we're not producing as many red blood cells as we could {another job our kidneys have}. Sure, adequate hydration may prevent these crystals, but just how much is adequate? After all, as CKD patients, we do have fluid restrictions.

As for actually causing kidney damage, yes, sulfa drugs can do that. As The National Kidney Foundation phrases it:

Other things that can damage the kidneys include kidney stones, urinary tract infections, and medications or drugs.

An allergic reaction to sulfa drugs can also cause kidney damage.

Allergies.About.Com reports:

People with sulfa allergy may also develop a type of hepatitis, and kidney failure, as a result of sulfa medications.

However, they are careful to point out that this is an uncommon reaction, occurring in less than 3% of users.

The antibiotics Bactrim and Septra are two of the most common sulfa drugs prescribed today. Most often, they'll be prescribed for a urinary tract or bladder infection. What makes it harder to pinpoint which drugs are sulfa drugs is that they don't always have 'sul' in their name.

That's also what makes it so important for you to impress upon your physician that you

1. do have CKD and
2. will not be taking any sulfa drugs

Wearing a medical alert bracelet might help you remember to be downright insistent that you will NOT be taking any sulfa drugs. The emergency room doctor did try to speak with my nephrologist before prescribing the drug for me, but couldn't get through… a situation we're all familiar with. He was not a specialist and made a judgment call that sulfa drugs would be all right for me.

Yet, when I finally got a response to my own calls to the nephrologist, he was horrified. This guy was not an emotional man so this really put me into a panic, especially since CKD was so new to me and I didn't really know the rules yet.

Number Three on the List

7/28/14 " Other studies have suggested that once diagnosed with kidney disease, weight loss may slow kidney disease progression, but this is the first research study to support losing belly fat and limiting phosphorus consumption as a possible way to prevent kidney disease from developing. Dr. Joseph Vassalotti, chief medical officer at the National Kidney Foundation 11/3/13"

Why has this little gem not caused more positive uproar? We already accept that high blood pressure and diabetes are the two leading causes of Chronic Kidney Disease and that preventing each may lessen your chances of developing the disease. Are we now looking at a third deterrent to developing CKD?

When I first wrote **What Is It and How Did I Get It? Early Stage Chronic Kidney Disease,** I was so eager to spread the word that I called Dr. Vassalotti and asked him to read the book. He was encouraging, and oh-so-willing to discuss anything CKD. I immediately trusted and believed what he had to say... and believe him now, especially with the research studies behind him.

So what is phosphorous, anyway? I defined it in my first book as:

One of the electrolytes, works with calcium for bone formation, but too much can cause calcification where you don't want it: joints, eyes, skin and heart.

Hmmm, I don't see any relation to preventing CKD there. I researched my usual sites and found that they also discussed the effects of phosphorus on the bones in CKD, but nothing about how limiting it might prevent the disease from developing.

Here's what I found about phosphorus at MedlinePlus, a service of the U.S. National Library of Medicine at The National Institutes of Health:

It plays an important role in how the body uses carbohydrates and fats. It is also needed for the body to make protein for the growth, maintenance, and repair of cells and tissues.

This is new information to me and makes sense. So we're not just dealing with phosphorus's importance in bone health, but in the body's use of carbs and fats.

If phosphorus is not doing its job as an electrolyte, there's a good chance you are gaining weight. Think about all those carbs and fats not properly being eliminated from your body. More caloric intake equals fat development. {I do realize we're not taking exercise into account here.}

This sentence from The Huffington Post's Healthy Living section last March caught my attention in a big way:

Belly fat is also much more inflammatory than fat located elsewhere in the body and can create its own inflammatory chemicals (as a tumor would).

Inflammatory? Isn't CKD an inflammatory disease? I went to The National Center for Biotechnology Information, which took me to the National Library of Medicine and finally to a National Institute of Health study for the answer:

The persistent inflammatory state is common in diabetes and Chronic Kidney Disease (CKD).

This is a lot to take in at once. What it amounts to is that another way to possibility prevent the onset of CKD is to lower your phosphorous intake so that you don't accumulate belly fat. All we need to know now is how this possible inflammatory state can cause CKD.

Thank you to Medical News Today for making it clear in this article:

The researchers from Johns Hopkins claim that reducing your waist circumference and cutting down on dietary phosphorus have been linked to lower levels of protein in the urine (albuminuria). The presence of this protein in urine is one of the first indicators of kidney disease.

I exercise. I follow the kidney diet. What was I eating before I developed CKD that might have contributed to its onset? Although I considered myself a health nut, I loved chocolate...milk chocolate. Yep, high in phosphorus.

As I researched different sites, I realized being a health nut was exactly the opposite of what I should have been. All of the following are on the majority of high phosphorous food lists: quinoa, oats, bran, milk, cheese, whole wheat, whole grain, dried beans or peas, brown rice or wild rice. If you're identifying with me, do not – I repeat do not – beat yourself up. Remember the connection between high phosphorous levels, belly fat, and CKD is new information.

Here's a hint: avoid processed foods since they have phosphorous added to extend their shelf life. I learned that somewhere along the way in my CKD journey, probably from my renal nutritionist. You can also add a recent product, flavored water, to the list of high phosphorous foods to avoid.

Unfortunately, phosphorous is not usually listed on labels. Although, I did see PHOS listed once or twice. Hopefully, it will become common usage to list phosphorous in the near future.

Awwww, Do I Have To?

8/4/14 That, ladies and gentlemen, is my internal dialogue every day when it's time to exercise… except when my exercise for the day is the dance lesson at Sustainable Blues.

My answer to myself is inevitably a resounding, YES!!! Okay, I know I have Chronic Kidney Disease – still holding at stage 3, thank you very much – and need to exercise to slow down the progression of the disease. But why? I mean, how does that help?

I'm going to quote heavily from **What Is It and How Did I Get It? Early Stage Chronic Kidney Disease** here. I've already done the research to answer the question but, quite frankly, have forgotten what I found. It's in the book.

Got your digital edition pulled up on your reading device so you can do a phrase search? Great. For those using the print version of the book {OMG, I feel like I'm teaching college again.}, let's turn to page 100 in *Chapter 10: Getting the Necessary Exercise.*

I knew exercise was important to control my weight. It would also improve my blood pressure and lower my cholesterol and triglyceride levels. The greater your triglycerides, the greater the risk of increasing your creatinine. There were other benefits, too, although you didn't have to have CKD to enjoy them: better sleep, and improved muscle function and strength. But, as with everything else you do that might impinge upon your health, check with your doctor before you start. I researched, researched and researched again. Each explanation of what exercise does for the body was more complicated than the last one I read. Keeping it simple, basically, there's a compound released by voluntary muscle contraction. It tells the body to repair itself and grow stronger. The idea is to start exercising slowly and then intensify your activity.

Yikes! There are some terms there those of you without the book may not know. Here's a little glossary for you.

Blood pressure: the pressure exerted by the blood against the walls of blood vessels. Blood pressure depends on the strength of the heartbeat, thickness and volume of the blood, the elasticity of the artery walls, and general health. {Encarta Dictionary}

Cholesterol: while the basis for both sex hormones and bile, can cause blockages if it accumulates in the lining of a blood vessel. {***What Is It and How Did I Get It? Early Stage Chronic Kidney Disease***}

Creatinine: chemical waste product that's produced by our muscle metabolism and to a smaller extent by eating meat. {MayoClinic.org}

Triglycerides: a type of fat found in your blood. Too much of this type of fat may raise the risk of coronary artery disease, especially in women. {Medline Plus}

I've used different sources for the definitions so as to bring you the most easily understood ones. After all, we're not doctors here.

Okay, I get it. Exercise is absolutely necessary since CKD prevents your body from adequately filtering wastes – like creatinine – from itself. Now my task was to find more exercise that I don't mind doing... like blues dancing. Even though I seem to be dancing at half-time, I come out of the bar thoroughly soaked despite the air conditioning. That's my personal indicator for effective exercise.

We went to the gun range yesterday. Later, on a whim, I started playing with the internet to see if target shooting burned enough calories to be considered exercise.

Whoopee! It does! It burns almost as many calories as half an hour on the stationary bike and uses a whole bunch of different muscles. Don't believe me? Take a look at the calorie counter at FitDay. Oh goody, another exercise I enjoy.

I have to admit that I enjoy the stationary bike, too, IF one of 'my' shows is on TV or I have a good book. I'm wondering how long I can do this type of exercise, though, since my knees have started declaring their presence in a demanding, non-loving way. Enter knee supports.

And, yes, I still do the Leslie Sansone Walking Tapes I described in My first book, but you've got to remember that your body becomes accustomed to a certain kind of exercise and then it isn't as effective anymore… and I was wearing knee supports for this, too.

I do the water walking I wrote about a few blogs back {No knee supports necessary.} as often as I can. Of course, no sooner did I decide I liked it then monsoon season started here. It's certainly not as bad as it's been in years past, but I'm still not going into a pool when there's rain. And then, there are the haboobs {dust storms}. No thanks, I'll find some kind of indoor exercise if there's a warning for one of those.

By the way, we are not alone in exercising more. We may do it because we have to, but the whole country is interested in exercising lately. According to the Centers for Disease Control and Prevention eNews headline of 5/15/14,

Neighborhood Support of Physical Activity on the Rise

What If You Don't Go?

8/11/14   We just got back from New York, which included stays in three different places. Only one- my buddy's pied `a terre in Brooklyn had a private bath… one bathroom for the two of us. In my niece's house on Long Island, we shared two bathrooms with two other adults and four children. In Manhattan, we shared two baths with twenty other tourists. This didn't exactly make for instant bathroom use when you needed it.

To add insult to injury, I've grown *very* accustomed to Arizona's immaculate public bathrooms with automatic faucets, flushes, soap dispensers, and towels. Let's just say New York has quite a bit of room for improvement in this area. The end result was that I didn't use the facilities as often as I needed to.

And I started wondering… what happens to the urine you don't void?

First things first, according to National Kidney and Urologic Diseases Information Clearinghouse (NKUDIC), A service of the National Institute of Diabetes and Digestive and Kidney Diseases (NIDDK), National Institutes of Health (NIH):

The amount of urine a person produces depends on many factors, such as the amounts of liquid and food a person consumes and the amount of fluid lost through sweat and breathing.

It was New York; it was not only hot, it was humid. I was drinking my allotted 64 ounces of liquid daily. I was breathing – as usual – and I was sweating quite a bit. Of course, I was eating, too.

In ***What Is It and How Did I Get It? Early Stage Kidney Disease***, I explained that:

Ingested food and liquid are digested in the stomach and bowels, and then absorbed in the blood. A renal artery carries the blood waste and water to the kidneys while a renal vein carries the filtered and sieved waste from the kidneys…..Additional important jobs of the kidneys are removing liquid waste from your body and balancing the minerals in the body. The two liquid waste products are urea which has been broken down from protein by the digestive system and creatinine which is a byproduct of muscle activity.

The problem with unregulated minerals such as sodium and potassium is that these minerals are needed to remain healthy but too much in the bloodstream becomes toxic. The kidneys remove these toxins and change them into urine that enters the bladder via the ureter…. Below the bladder is the urethra, the passage to the outside of your body. This is, of course, a highly simplified explanation. The toxins would build up and poison you if the kidneys were damaged.

This is right at the beginning of the book on pages 2 and 3.

Now that we know how it works, we can go back to my original question: What if you don't urinate when your bladder is full?

Well, maybe we should explore the bladder a bit more. WebMD tells us the following about the bladder.

The bladder stores urine, allowing urination to be infrequent and voluntary. The bladder is lined by layers of muscle tissue that stretch to accommodate urine. The normal capacity of the bladder is 400 to 600 mL. During urination, the bladder muscles contract, and two sphincters (valves) open to allow urine to flow out. Urine exits the bladder into the urethra, which carries urine out of the body.

So, there I was with a full bladder and my body telling me to empty it, but I didn't. What happened to the urine?

It's time to mention that the ureters don't have any way to stop the urine flowing back into the kidneys if you don't void. There are two sphincters at the bottom of your bladder leading into the urethra, but you can only voluntarily control one of them.

Interesting fact: the urethra is longer in men because it passes through the penis. Sorry fact: because our urethras are shorter, we women are more prone to urinary tract infections.

Uh-oh, urine was moving back into my poor, already compromised kidneys. This urine flow back could further damage the capillaries and tubules making them even less effective at filtering my blood. The kidney's pelvis and calyces – their central collection region – might become dilated, causing hydronephrosis. Or I might end up with a kidney infection from the bacteria forced back in. This is called pyelonephritis.

Hang on there. I'm going to use the Merriam-Webster Medical dictionary for some definitions here.

CALYX (*plural* ca·lyx·es *or* ca·ly·ces *also* ca·li·ces): a cuplike division of the renal pelvis surrounding one or more renal papillae

CAPILLARY a: resembling a hair especially in slender elongated form
            b: having a very small bore

HYDRONEPHROSIS: cystic distension of the kidney caused by the accumulation of urine in the renal pelvis as a result of obstruction to outflow and accompanied by atrophy of the kidney structure and cyst formation

RENAL PAPILLA: the apex of a renal pyramid which projects into the lumen of a calyx of the kidney and through which collecting tubules discharge urine

RENAL PELVIS: a funnel-shaped structure in each kidney that is formed at one end by the expanded upper portion of the ureter lying in the renal sinus and at the other end by the union of the calyxes of the kidney

TUBULE: a small tube; *especially*: a slender elongated anatomical channel

But, wait before you get all excited about the damage I've done to myself – or worse, yourself - you should know it would take a tremendous amount of flow back before any of this happens. Be aware of your urge to urinate, follow through if you can, and don't worry if you can't every once in a while {but remember that I'm not a doctor}. And I wonder why I've felt the urge to urinate the whole time I've been writing today's blog.

Facebook and CKD

8/18/14   I'm lucky. I have plenty of support here from Bear, the daughters, the almost sons-in-law, and the neighbors. But many people don't have others to talk to. That's why I'll be writing about online support groups today.

The blog has a major presence on Facebook. That started with the administrator's invitation to join **P2P, {Peer To Peer} – Support for The Chronically Ill and Friends & Family** several years ago.

This is a closed group of 6,198 members with invitation by email. As with most closed groups, the idea is for the members to be able to freely discuss whatever troubles them. I've also noticed lots of support for other than illness issues here… and loads of sharing happinesses.

Although I do not have a transplant, shortly after **What Is It and How Did I Get It? Early Stage Chronic Kidney Disease** was published, the administrators asked me to post this weekly blog on **The Transplant Community Outreach's** page under the heading KIDNEY MATTERS. I remember trying to dissuade them from this idea since I only knew about early stage, but they were adamant… and I'm still posting the blog there. This is a public support page with 5,633 members. I've received a number of comments indicating that all stages of CKD patients are welcome.

Then there's **The Renal Patient Support Group** {RPSG} Facebook & BlogSpot, another closed group, with 5,305 members. I find this group extremely interactive concerning rides, requests for new information, and information about local treatment centers that you won't find elsewhere. Their administrator has added a link to this blog on their page.

Chronic Kidney Disease, End Stage Renal Failure is a smaller {71 members} closed group. It is quite homey and inviting. When I go there, I feel like I'm visiting my neighbor. That doesn't mean it's not worthwhile, though. Sometimes you need that homey feel to understand what you're reading.

Kidney Disease, Diet Ideas, and Help 1 with 7,611 members is another closed group. You can usually like a closed group to join or inbox the administrator. This is how they describe the group:

This is a closed, private group run by genuine Kidney patients for people with Kidney Disease including Dialysis to Transplant also for Carers to be able to offer and receive their support and knowledge in complete privacy from your friends on Facebook, to cover all aspects including discussing openly and sharing ideas on how each of our members is coping , how it affects us in day to day living, medications, side effects also their Diets, Drinks and lifestyle in accordance to our individual requirements and to also share ideas and recipes for CKD. ALWAYS SEEK MEDICAL ADVICE BEFORE TRYING ANYTHING NEW.

All the Facebook support groups remind you they are not doctors. It is important for you to remember that so you check with your nephrologist before trying anything new. Better safe than sorry. Notice, too, that most support groups welcome family, friends, caregivers, and others somehow involved with the kidney disease patient. The groups usually do not discriminate, but welcome all who are interested.

One of the newer groups is *Women's Renal Failure Support Group*, a closed group with 579 members. There is a free give and take about {Surprise!} specifically women's issues. While I'm post-menopausal myself, I find I especially enjoy the younger women's posts about whether and if they can become pregnant, the hints and advice they give each other, and their generous support along this difficult journey for CKD sufferers.

People of Color Renal, Kidney, Dialysis, and Transplant Support is not restricted to people of color, although there are many posts that deal specifically with this group of particularly at risk for CKD people. It is a closed group with 207 members. I think the administrator nails the problem with reaching minorities in his description:

People of Color Renal, Kidney, Dialysis and Transplant Support Group is for sharing information on people who are close to renal failure, dialysis or on dialysis or who have had a kidney transplant in the hopes of educating and offering support. Renal failure is the most prevalent among the minority communities but they are the least informed with options of dealing with this epidemic. This group is just not for minorities only but for all concerned with End Stage Renal Disease.

By the way, the key word in all these support groups is *sharing*. There are many other groups I post in because I feel they are so worthwhile in their efforts to educate CKD sufferers by sharing information AND by allowing them to vent, question, rant, and – of course – providing an opportunity for their members to support each other.

Some of the others are: **GM Kidney Information Network, Kidney disease isn't for sissies, Kidney Disease is Not a Joke Group, KidneysRus** {Not an organ selling site. This is illegal in the U.S.}, **UK Kidney Support, National Kidney Foundation, Canadian Kidney Connection, and The Bhutan Kidney Foundation**.

I know I've left out some really good support sites, but I'll plead lack of space. Some of the foreign sites are excellent and it's fun to see how they deal with CKD differently than we do in the U.S. Well, maybe my sense of fun is different from yours, but I enjoy it.

Never NSAIDS

8/25/14   Never what? One of the first rules we learn as Chronic Kidney Disease patients is never to take a NSAID, a non-steroidal anti-inflammatory drug. Raise your hand if you remember why.

Hello fellow with the beard in the back of the room; what do you say? Correct! They further damage the kidneys. Can you tell us how? No? Don't feel bad. Most people can't, even those suffering from CKD.

What was that? Oh, you want over the counter (non-prescription) names of some NSAIDS? Sure. Here's a list courtesy of Nsaids-list.

- Aspirin (Aspirin is a brand name; the chemical is called acetylsalicylic acid)
- Celecoxib (Celebrex)
- Dexdetoprofen (Keral)
- Diclofenac (Voltaren, Cataflam, Voltaren-XR)
- Diflunisal (Dolobid)
- Etodolac (Lodine, Lodine XL)
- Etoricoxib (Algix)
- Fenoprofen (Fenopron, Nalfron)
- Firocoxib (Equioxx, Previcox)
- Flurbiprofen (Urbifen, Ansaid, Flurwood, Froben)
- Ibuprofen (Advil, Brufen, Motrin, Nurofen, Medipren, Nuprin)
- Indomethacin (Indocin, Indocin SR, Indocin IV)
- Ketoprofen (Actron, Orudis, Oruvail, Ketoflam)
- Ketorolac (Toradol, Sprix, Toradol IV/IM, Toradol IM)
- Licofelone (under development)
- Lornoxicam (Xefo)
- Loxoprofen (Loxonin, Loxomac, Oxeno)
- Lumiracoxib (Prexige)
- Meclofenamic acid (Meclomen)
- Mefenamic acid (Ponstel)
- Meloxicam (Movalis, Melox, Recoxa, Mobic)
- Nabumetone (Relafen)
- Naproxen (Aleve, Anaprox, Midol Extended Relief, Naprosyn, Naprelan)
- Nimesulide (Sulide, Nimalox, Mesulid)

- Oxaporozin (Daypro, Dayrun, Duraprox)
- Parecoxib (Dynastat)
- Piroxicam (Feldene)
- Rofecoxib (Vioxx, Ceoxx, Ceeoxx)
- Salsalate (Mono-Gesic, Salflex, Disalcid, Salsitab)
- Sulindac (Clinoril)
- Tenoxicam (Mobiflex)
- Tolfenamic acid (Clotam Rapid, Tufnil)
- Valdecoxib (Bextra)
-

Yes, young lady in the third row. This is a bit more detailed a list than you'd expected? Okay, let's go back to **What Is It and How Did I Get It? Early Stage Chronic Kidney Disease** for a simple explanation of NSAID. Please turn to page 134. Those of you with digital copies of the book, search the phrase. Everyone have it?

NSAID: Non-steroidal anti-inflammatory drugs such as ibuprofen, aspirin, Aleve or naproxen usually used for arthritis or pain management, can worsen kidney disease, sometimes irreversibly.

So now we're back to the original question. How *do* NSAIDS further damage our kidneys?

By the way, as early as 1984, the National Institutes of Health published a journal article from the Canadian Medical Association Journal entitled *Adverse effects of NSAIDs on renal function*.

Why no, I'm not procrastinating at all. Here's the answer to today's question. I found this explanation at a site that's new to me – empower.com:

All NSAIDs work by blocking the action of cyclooxygenase (COX). This enzyme performs a key step in the synthesis of prostaglandins {Me here with a definition of this word from the freedictionary.com – a group of potent hormone like substances that produce a wide range of body response such as changing capillary permeability, smooth muscle tone, clumping of platelets,and endocrine and exocrine functions. They are involved in the pain process of inflammation.} which produce many effects in the body. Two of the effects are pain and inflammation for injured tissue. Other effects include protection of the stomach and homeostasis (regulation) of kidney function. The COX enzyme comes in two forms, COX-1 and COX-2. For a while, it was thought that COX-2 produces the pain and inflammation prostaglandins, while COX-1 produces the protective and regulatory prostaglandins

.

That's right, NSAIDS interfere with the regulation of the kidney function. How? Another good question from the middle of the room. According to the National Kidney Foundation:

...because they reduce the blood flow to the kidney.

So now we need to know why blood flow to the kidneys is important for CKD patients. If you look at a picture of your kidney, you'll see that blood with wastes in it is brought to the kidneys by the renal artery and clean blood is exited from the kidneys by the renal vein. Your kidneys are already compromised which means they are not doing such a great job of filtering your blood.

Reduce the blood flow and you're exacerbating the problem you already have... and all you need to do is avoid NSAIDS to avoid this problem. You're right, class, that's not exactly true, but it will help you preserve more of your kidney function.

Any questions for me? For each other? Well then, thank you for being such a willing and involved group of students.

While we all know this isn't really a classroom and I'm not a doctor, this should answer a great many of the questions I've received via email or comments.

Laboring on Labor Day

9/1/14 Today is Labor Day. We celebrate it every year. But what is it? This holiday, first celebrated in New York City in 1885 or even 1882, was founded to celebrate workers and their contributions to society. In other words, we're celebrating – just as the name suggests – labor.

We, as Chronic Kidney Disease patients, also labor… every day of the year, every year of our lives. We cannot contribute to society unless we labor to save ourselves. Just keep that in the back of your mind as you bar-b-que, watch a parade, or go to a picnic today. Maybe it'll help you stick to your renal diet, if nothing else.

Our community, our families, and our doctors labor for us, too. So do researchers. You may remember a reader's comment back in July about *the New England Journal of Medicine*. One of the review articles in the journal concerned Acute Kidney Injury (AKI) and Chronic Kidney Disease (CKD).

On the very first page of **What Is It and How Did I Get It? Early Stage Chronic Kidney Disease**, I wrote:

…chronic is not acute. It means long term, whereas acute usually means quick onset and short duration.

All those years of teaching English in high school and college paid off for me right there in that sentence.

I'd always thought that AKI and CKD were separate issues and I'll bet you did, too. But Dr. L.S. Chawla and his co-writers based the following conclusion on the labor of epidemiologists and others:

Chronic Kidney Disease is a risk factor for acute kidney injury, acute kidney injury is a risk factor for the development of Chronic Kidney Disease, and both acute kidney injury and Chronic Kidney Disease are risk factors for cardiovascular disease.

I keep wondering why this article was published on Independence Day, but maybe I'm trying to make too much of that. You know, independence from ignorance about new findings concerning our disease, that sort of thing.

Not surprisingly, the risk factors for AKI {Once again, that's acute kidney injury.} are the same as those for CKD… except for one peculiar circumstance. Having CKD itself can raise the risk of AKI 10 times. Whoa! If you're Black, of an advanced age {Hey!}, or have diabetes, you already know you're at risk for CKD, or are the one out of nine in our country that has it. Once you've developed CKD, you've just raised the risk for AKI 10 times. I'm getting a little nervous here.

Someone I grew up with just had AKI which temporarily shut his kidneys down. This was a month ago. While his kidneys are fully functioning now, because he had this episode, he's at risk for CKD and Cardiovascular Disease {CVD, as long as we're making a little no sodium alphabet soup here}.

It makes sense, as researchers and doctors are beginning to see, that these are all connected. I'm not a doctor or a researcher, but I can understand that if you've had some kind of insult to your kidney, it would be more apt to develop CKD.

And the CVD risk? Let's think of it this way. You've had AKI. That period of weakness in the kidneys opens them up to CKD. We already know there's a connection between CKD and CVD. Throw that AKI into the mix, and you have more of a chance to develop CVD whether or not you've had a problem in this area before.

Let's not go off the deep end here. If you've had AKI, you just need to be monitored to see if CKD develops and avoid nephrotoxic {kidney poisoning} medications such as NSAIDS – just wrote about those in last week's blog – , contrast dyes, and radioactive substances.

This is just so circular! It was nephrotoxic medication that caused AKI in the first place for the person I know.

As with CKD, your hypertension and diabetes {if you have them.} need to be monitored, too. Then there's the renal diet, especially low sodium foods. The kicker here is that no one knows if this is helpful in avoiding

CKD after an AKI… it's a 'just in case' kind of thing to help ward off any CKD and possible CVD from the CKD.

Has your primary care doctor recommended a daily low dose aspirin with your nephrologist's approval? This is to protect your heart against CVD since you already have CKD which raises the risk of CVD. Now here's where it gets confusing, the FDA has recently revoked its endorsement of such a regiment.

Sometimes, you need to just sit down and have a heart to heart, or more realistically leave a message with your concerns, with your PCP {Primary Care Physician} and talk it out.

It's All Connected

9/8/14   I got a call from my primary care physician telling me that while I had improved my BUN, Creatinine, BUN/Creatinine Ratio, LDL, and eGFR levels on my last blood test, the Microalbumin, Urine, Random value was abnormal at 17.3. I checked my results on the practice's website to make certain I had heard her correctly.

When I finally finished congratulating myself for all these improvements, I started to question why the Microalbuminuria value was out of range. I knew it hadn't been out of range last year, but I did have Chronic Kidney Disease. That in itself would have meant it would be out of whack, wouldn't it?

Here we go again. I pulled out my trusty copy of ***What Is It and How Did I Get It? Early Stage Chronic Kidney Disease*** and turned to *Chapter 5: What Flows Through You,* The Random Urine Tests, number 9299 on page 52 and found:

tests for micro, or very small amounts, of albumin in the urine. Ur stands for urine. Albumin is a form of protein that is water soluble. Urine is a liquid, a form of water, so the albumin should have been dissolved. Protein in the urine may be an indication of kidney disease.

Of course I wanted more. We all know micro from micro-mini skirts {Are you old enough to remember those?} and microscope.

Wait, if protein in the urine "may be an indication of kidney disease" – which I have – why was this a problem? Or was it a problem?

Both high blood pressure {which I do have} and diabetes {which I don't} could be the cause since both may lead to the proteinuria {protein in the urine; albumin is a protein as mentioned above.} which may indicate CKD. Microalbuminuria could be the first step to proteinuria.

But, as usual with medical conditions, it's not that black and white. I scurried over to our old friend WebMD to look for other risk factors and found these.
- Obesity
- Age over 65

- Family history of kidney disease
- Preeclampsia (high blood pressure and proteinuria in pregnancy)
- Race and ethnicity: African-Americans, Native Americans, Hispanics, and Pacific Islanders are more likely than whites to have high blood pressure and develop kidney disease and proteinuria.

While I'm well past child bearing, I'm also over 65 and, ummm, clinically obese. Does that mean proteinuria is to be my new norm?

Maybe there's something more I can do about this. According to the U.S. Department of Health and Human Services' National Kidney and Urologic Diseases' Information Clearinghouse (NKUDIC):

In addition to blood glucose and blood pressure control, the National Kidney Foundation recommends restricting dietary salt and protein. A doctor may refer a patient to a dietitian to help develop and follow a healthy eating plan.

 This is nuts! I have CKD. I already restrict myself to five ounces of protein a day. I've abolished table salt from the house and watch the salt content in the foods I eat. I'm handling my blood pressure with Losartan/HCTZ. {See the next paragraph.} I haven't progressed from microalbuminuria to proteinuria, yet I'm still doing more damage to my body.

MedicineNet explains the Losartan/HCTZ very well:

Losartan (more specifically, the chemical formed when the **liver** converts the inactive losartan into an active chemical) blocks the angiotensin receptor. By blocking the action of angiotensin, losartan relaxes the muscles, dilates blood vessels and thereby reduces blood pressure....Hydrochlorothiazide (HCTZ) is a diuretic (water pill) used for treating high blood pressure (hypertension) and accumulation of fluid. It works by blocking salt and fluid reabsorption in the kidneys, causing an increased amount of urine containing salt (diuresis).

Uh-oh, that leaves blood glucose, which has never been high for me. However, my A1C has been high since this whole CKD ride has started.

Let's backtrack a little. The Mayo Clinic tells us:

The A1C test result reflects your average blood sugar level for the past two to three months. Specifically, the A1C test measures what percentage of your hemoglobin — a protein in red blood cells that carries oxygen — is coated with sugar (glycated). The higher your A1C level, the poorer your blood sugar control and the higher your risk of diabetes complications.

I don't have diabetes…yet. It's becoming clear that I will – in addition to worsening my CKD – if I don't pay even more attention to my diet and become more stringent about exercising. It's sooooo easy to say not today when the arthritis rears its ugly head…or knee.

It's been said there's no way to do it, but to do it {By me, folks. Ask my children.} So now I need to take my own advice and get back to the stricter enforcement of the rules I know I need to live by. After all, they let me live.

If you ever needed proof that the body is an intricate thing with all its part being integrated, you got it today.

From Deficiency to Support

9/15/14   I went to a birthday party in a hotel I've been interested in since we moved to Arizona. It was nice, but what was nicer was sitting next to a young friend who happens to be a ball player.

We both ordered vegetarian dishes. He knows I have Chronic Kidney Disease and started talking about my renal diet… and the limitation of five ounces of protein per day. "Don't you worry about protein deficiency?" he asked with alarm.

And that got me to thinking. According to The Centers for Disease Control and Prevention, as a woman above the age of 19 and all the way up to beyond the age of 70, I need 46 grams of protein a day.
Well, how many grams are in an ounce? I went directly to AskNumbers.com for the answer. While I'm not innumerate, I don't have the patience for long, involved mathematical formulations. That's where I found both a convenient ounce to gram conversion calculator and a conversion chart.

According to the site:

5 Ounces = 141.7476155 Grams

That's way more than the 46 grams of protein required by a woman my age. So what was my friend concerned about?

Men in the same age range need 56 grams of protein as I saw on the CDC site mentioned above. That's still only 1.9753418664 ounces. This wasn't making any sense to me.

I went right back to **What Is It and How Did I Get It? Early Stage Chronic Kidney Disease** for the definition of protein:

Amino acids arranged in chains joined by peptide bonds to form a compound, important because some proteins are hormones, enzymes, and antibodies.

I decided it wasn't as important to know what they were as it was to know what they do. I found the definition for hormones in my first book:

Gland produced chemicals that trigger tissues to do whatever their particular job is.

Got it! Sort of like a catalyst to get those tissues working.

I went to Dictionary.com for the medical definition of enzyme:

Any of numerous proteins or conjugated proteins produced by living oganisms and functioning as specialized catalysts for biochemical reactions.

There's that word 'catalyst' again.

Well, what about antibodies? Using the same source, I found this:

 A protein substance produced in the blood or tissues in response to a specific antigen, such as a bacterium or a toxin, that destroys or weakens bacteria and neutralizes organic poisons, thus forming the basis of immunity.

Lots of definitions here, but the important part is that they all explain how important protein intake is. I think my friend's error was not in worrying about protein deficiency, but in getting the math confused. I thank him for his concern nonetheless.

Moving right along…some readers have asked for online support groups that are not on Facebook since they – these particular readers – aren't. I've also included telephone and face to face support groups since I know some of you receive the blog when someone with a computer prints it out to give to you. Please remember these are not recommendations. Some I know and am comfortable with; others are new to me.

Lori Hartwell's **Renal Support Network** offers monthly support groups.

American Association of Kidney Patients (AAKP) offers a listing of support groups by state at. Not all states are listed. These are in person meetings.

The National Kidney Foundation (NKF) has peer matching telephone support. You will need to be interviewed first. You can find more information on their website. You can also call 855-653-7337 (855-NKF-PEER) toll free or email nkfcares@kidney.org to participate.

For my Australian readers, you can join a ***Kidney Club*** by emailing kidneyhelponline@kidney.org.au or free call 1800 454 363.

There are even ***Meetup Groups*** for CKD patients.

The more I researched, the more I realized that each state, and even each city, in the U.S. has their own groups. I gather it's the same in other countries. If none of these is what you're looking for, I'd suggest an online search for CKD support groups in your area.

Sleepus Interruptus

9/22/14   I just started – and trashed – three different versions of what I thought today's blog would be about because I didn't understand the research. That's the trouble with not being a doctor, and why I always remind you to speak with your nephrologist before you take anyone's advice about your Chronic Kidney Disease, even mine.

I finally decided to write about my first choice. This is yet another indication that our hunches are right. My hunch after a night of waking up just about every hour was to write about CKD and interrupted sleep. I should have listened to myself and saved all that time.

DaVita tells us there are several reasons CKD patients have sleep problems.

- restless leg syndrome
- sleep apnea
- inadequate dialysis clearance
- emotions
- changes in sleep patterns
- caffeine

We share most of these reasons with those who do not have CKD except for those dealing with dialysis. This includes the inadequate dialysis clearance. It also includes restless leg syndrome which is usually associated with hemodialysis session. Since I only write about earlier stage, I won't be discussing these causes.

Let's talk about sleep apnea. I wrote a blog on August 12, 2012 that refers to this. The most important information from that blog is I found a study on Medscape.com which clearly links sleep apnea and hypertension.

"We think there may be a causative factor here; that sleep apnea may be causing direct glomerular injury," Dr. John J. Sim (Kaiser Permanente, Los Angeles, CA) told renal*wire* . "We already know that sleep apnea causes hypertension and that hypertension causes kidney disease." If some degree of causality can be shown, it's possible that treating sleep apnea may slow the progression of kidney disease, the authors speculate.

This particular study was conducted in 2005.

Obstructive sleep apnea (OSA) was also the subject of January 13, 2014's blog. That's where the following information is from.

Have I ever told you I have sleep apnea? And that this affects CKD patients? I do and it does. According to one of the National Institutes of Health's sites, sleep apnea can raise blood pressure, which in itself is one of the problems of CKD. It can also result in glomerular hyperfiltration. This is from a 2010 study.

Okay, so I have sleep apnea, had a sleep study and started wearing a Mandibular Advancement Device (MAD) at night to correct the problem, yet I still experience interrupted sleep.

Hmmm, what is this 'changes in sleep patterns'? Oh, of course. Because I have CKD, I become more tired and even drowsy during the day. Maybe I'll sit on the couch in the family room to read for a bit; maybe I'll even lay down there; and maybe – just maybe – I'll fall asleep during the day. Nothing wrong with naps, but if they're long naps they could interfere with your sleep pattern.

So can going to bed earlier. I tried that on really tired days and ended up waking up repeatedly. I do go right back to sleep, but it just didn't seem restful. Keep in mind that as you age, your sleep cycles are lighter and shorter. So I may think I'm getting all the sleep I need, but the waking up interrupts the cycling of the different stages of sleep and then I start the cycles all over again.

WebMD tells us:

During the deep stages of NREM sleep, the body repairs and regenerates tissues, builds bone and muscle, and appears to strengthen the immune system. As you get older, you sleep more lightly and get less deep sleep. Aging is also associated with shorter time spans of sleep, although studies show the amount of sleep needed doesn't appear to diminish with age.

Uh-oh, the deep stages of NREM {non-rapid eye movement} sleep are stages 3 and 4 which I may be missing by constantly waking up. These are also the stages during which the body restores itself.

Going back to DaVita's list, I can see that emotions might cause a sleep issue. I dwell on the family's medical problems, or someone I know and love who is out of work, or even my sweet Bella's brush with cancer and I can get myself truly worked up. So I don't. I mean I don't think about these things at bedtime. If I can't seem to get them out of my head, I write a list of things to think about tomorrow. As simplistic as it sounds, it works for me. This is one piece of advice you don't need to check with your nephrologist.

Wait a minute! Who included my beloved caffeine on this list??????
This is where I get emotional. Those two cups of caffeine a day are the only item on my renal diet that help me not feel deprived. Okay, maybe we do need to be a bit rational about this

This is what The National Sleep Foundation has to offer us about caffeine and sleep:

Caffeine enters the bloodstream through the stomach and small intestine and can have a stimulating effect as soon as 15 minutes after it is consumed. Once in the body, caffeine will persist for several hours: it takes about 6 hours for one half of the caffeine to be eliminated.

Six hours for only half to be eliminated? You mean, twelve hours for all of it to be eliminated? I have got to stop drinking caffeine after noon. Okay, I can learn to live with that. Heck, it's better than no coffee at all.

Hopefully these suggestions will take care of my interrupted sleep problems. Now what about yours? Remember to speak with your nephrologist if you want to explore any of my suggestions. As far as the emotions causing sleep problems, if my trick doesn't work for you and you feel you need professional help with your emotions, please get it.

Oh, the Pressure!

9/29/14   I was surprised to discover that The Tubac Presidio State Historic Park is manned by a staff of volunteers – except for their director. That got me to thinking about the pressure they all must be under... which got me to thinking about pressure of all kinds and its effect on blood pressure.

Not only have I written about blood pressure in **What Is It and How Did I Get It? Early Stage Chronic Kidney Disease**, but also in several blogs. So why write about the same topic again, you ask? This time, I took a look at how to take your blood pressure and some of the machines on the market.

Have I ever told you that when I am at my sleep apnea doctor's office, my blood pressure always starts at about 150/89? That's high and I tell them it's not my usual reading. We're way past the white coat syndrome {blood pressure rising simply because you're in a doctor's office.} here, so they take it again on the other arm and it's something about 110/72. I like that, but it's not my usual reading, either. Back to the first arm: 130/79. Bingo!

I asked my primary care physician why this happens and she asked me to describe the monitor they used. As I did, she started nodding her head. Apparently, this type of automatic blood pressure monitor is notorious for being incorrect... yet doctors still use it for its ease.

Then she asked me how they held my arm while taking my blood pressure and slowly shook her head as I answered. It seems there is a right way and a wrong way to hold the arm and – to further complicate matters – they differ depending upon the type of monitor being used. I went to WebMD for the following:

Before Checking Your Blood Pressure
- Find a quiet place to check your blood pressure. You will need to listen for your heartbeat.
- Make sure that you are comfortable and relaxed with a recently emptied bladder (a full bladder may affect your reading).
- Roll up the sleeve on your arm or remove any tight-sleeved clothing.

- Rest in a chair next to a table for 5 to 10 minutes. Your arm should rest comfortably at heart level. Sit up straight with your back against the chair, legs uncrossed. Rest your forearm on the table with the palm of your hand facing up.

Were you surprised as I was at the direction to empty your bladder? Think for a minute. Have any of your doctors requested you do that before they took your blood pressure reading? Yet, it makes sense. Not only will the full bladder itself affect the reading, so will the worry that you need to get to the restroom as soon as possible.

Okay, now we're ready. What's next? This time, I went to The Mayo Clinic:

- Check your monitor's accuracy.
- Measure your blood pressure twice daily. (Once in the morning before you take any medications, and once in the evening.)
- Don't measure your blood pressure right after you wake up.
- Avoid food, caffeine, tobacco and alcohol for 30 minutes before taking a measurement
- Don't talk while taking your blood pressure.

Whoa! This simple act of placing your arm, wrist, or finger in a monitor is not simple at all when you break it down into smaller elements. I admit it; I'm a talker and have been told a time or two to stop talking while my blood pressure is being measured.

I also like to get my chores out of the way as soon as I wake up, but I see I can't. This makes for a long morning routine for me. First I take off the wrist braces I wear at night for the neuropathy. Then I clean the mandibular advancement appliance I've had in my mouth all night for the sleep apnea and brush it and my teeth. Usually I would drink that delicious first cup of coffee now, but if I do, I have to wait for 30 minutes before taking my blood pressure. Hmmm, I have to wait 15 minutes to use the bite rim to readjust my mandibular anyway. But where do I fit in the medications? Oh, I'll work it out.

Well, what about the different kinds of blood pressure monitors? I use a wrist monitor which my PCP is simply not thrilled with. Her feeling is that I'm taking my pressure through two bones, the radius and the ulna, as opposed to only one bone, the humerus, with an arm device. There's also the finger monitor, but that could be a problem if you have thin or cold fingers.

There are manual and battery operated versions of these monitors. If you use an arm monitor, be aware that larger cuffs are available if needed. The one thing most blood pressure sites agree upon is that it's not a good idea to rely on drugstore monitors for your readings.

Most doctors will agree that the old fashioned sphygmomanometer is the best. You'll find this defined on page 135 of ***What Is It and How Did I Get It? Early Stage Chronic Kidney Disease***:

The cuff, the measuring device and the wires that connect the two in a machine used to measure your blood pressure, commonly called a blood pressure meter.

I find myself wanting to make some crack about writing this blog raising my blood pressure, but in all honesty, writing the blog is still one of my joys.

The Way I See It

10/6/14   There I sat moping because my eyes are getting worse and I didn't know why. So I did what I do best {and what brings me right up again, believe it or not.} and started researching. I found multiple answers! That's terrific because I've already drunk my two cups of coffee today, so I couldn't turn to them for solace.

You've probably figured out the answers are mostly Chronic Kidney Disease related. This is not something I wrote about in ***What Is It and How Did I Get It? Early Stage Chronic Kidney Disease***. When I researched for the book, macular degeneration never even peeked out at me. {How do you like that play on vision related words? Macular – peeked? No? Oh well.}

Anyway…. let's do our usual back to the basics for a topic we haven't visited in a while. Macular degeneration is:

An eye disease that progressively destroys the macula, the central portion of the retina, impairing central vision. Macular degeneration rarely causes total blindness because only the center of vision is affected

This is according to MedicineNet.

I suppose the part about not causing total blindness should make me feel better, but I need more information first. The retina? Anyone? No? It's:

… a multi-layered sensory tissue that lines the back of the eye. It contains millions of photoreceptors that capture light rays and convert them into electrical impulses. These impulses travel along the optic nerve to the brain where they are turned into images. There are two types of photoreceptors in the retina: rods and cones. The retina contains approximately 6 million cones. The cones are contained in the macula, the portion of the retina responsible for central vision. They are most densely packed within the fovea, the very center portion of the **macula**. Cones function best in bright light and allow us to appreciate color. There are approximately 125 million rods. They are spread throughout the peripheral retina and function best in dim lighting. The rods are responsible for peripheral and night vision.

I had to dig deep for a thorough, yet easily understood definition. Thank you St. Luke's Cataract and Laser Institute for helping out here.

Well, now you understand why I keep posting all those pictures containing glorious color. That's my way of saving up color for when I can't see it anymore. Although, it's really the rods that are causing me most trouble right now.

Dim the lighting and I can't tell what I'm looking at. I don't know where Bear is in a dim room unless he speaks and my poor black and white Bella! My dog's been walked into so often I don't know why she doesn't just run when she sees me coming.

However, it's not as easy as just that. There are two kinds of macular degeneration: wet and dry. I went back to our old pal The Mayo Clinic for the definitions:

Wet macular degeneration is a chronic eye disease that causes vision loss in the center of your field of vision. Wet macular degeneration is generally caused by abnormal blood vessels that leak fluid or blood into the region of the macula (MAK-u-luh). The macula is in the center of the retina (the layer of tissue on the inside back wall of your eyeball). Wet macular degeneration is one of two types of age-related macular degeneration. The other type — dry macular degeneration — is more common and less severe. Wet macular degeneration almost always begins as dry macular degeneration. It's not clear what causes wet macular degeneration.

Wait a minute. Did you catch that "age-related macular degeneration"? That's what I have and that's where the Chronic Kidney Disease comes into our equation.

I went to The National Institutes of Health website to find the conclusions from a *Journal of American Society of Nephrology* study about the relationship between macular degeneration and Chronic Kidney Disease:

...persons with moderate Chronic Kidney Disease were 3 times more likely to develop early age-related macular degeneration than persons with no/mild Chronic Kidney Disease.

Thank you very much, CKD, for another undesired gift. To be honest, although this has not shown up anywhere else in my family history, I don't know if I would have developed macular degeneration even if I didn't have CKD. Apparently, smoking is another risk factor and that is something I played around with for decades – never becoming a chain smoker, but smoking nervously and socially. Hey, we didn't really know what the consequences could be at that time.

WebMD tells us the other risk factors:

... high blood pressure, high cholesterol, obesity, and being light skinned, female, and having a light eye color are also risk factors for macular degeneration.

Un-oh, I fit every one of these criterion {if light brown eyes are considered light eye color}. Sometimes I wish I had foresight instead of hindsight. While I couldn't have done anything about my race, sex, or eye color, there's quite a bit I could have worked on as far as hypertension, hyperlipidemia, and weight.

Because I am a Pollyanna and need to find hope everywhere, my hope here is that my experience can at least serve as an object lesson for our younger Chronic Kidney Disease sufferers. Sort of a do-as-I-say, not do-as-I-do example, if you will.

Put your Back into It for a Few Minutes

10/13/14   You can always tell what's troubling me by the topic of each week's blog. This week it turns out I have "irritated disks." I kid you not. It actually makes sense since Bear has some ruptured disks that won't be treated until Friday and I've taken over his chores for a while.

Let's go back to the very beginning to explain this one. Here's the definition I'll be using for disk:

Fibrocartilaginous material between spinal vertebrae which provides a cushion-like support against shock.

Thank you, *McGraw-Hill Concise Dictionary of Modern Medicine* for that. Here we go again: a definition that needs another definition to understand the first definition.

Naturally you'd want to know what fibrocartilage is. According to *Gale Encyclopedia of Medicine*, it's:

Cartilage that consists of dense fibers.

Hang on there. We need one more definition. I went to MedicineNet for this definition of cartilage:

….It is a firm tissue but is softer and much more flexible than bone. So we have soft, firm, flexible, dense fiber material between our spinal vertebrae.

Our what? Vertebrae is:

a bone of the spinal column, typically consisting of a thick body, a bony arch enclosing a hole for the spinal cord, and stubby projections that connect with adjacent bones.

For the definition of spinal column {And you thought we were done with definitions.}, I chose to use *Collins Dictionary*:

A series of contiguous or interconnecting bony or cartilaginous segments that surround and protect the spinal cord.

I used to tell my children when they were little and my back hurt that the stuff between my vertebrae that acts as a cushion wasn't cushioning right. Simple, direct, and to the point. Apparently I'm on the verge of that again. And I WILL stop it before it gets any worse.

How, you ask? My chiropractor suggested ice for twenty minutes, then take it off for an hour and repeat... and repeat... and repeat. With Chronic Kidney Disease, I *need* the daily exercise to keep my organs – all of them – strong, especially since CKD can eventually affect your other organs. It's our not-quite-filtered blood that feeds these organs, so we need to keep them healthy in as many ways as we can.

The icing is helping, but I have rediscovered my inability to do nothing for twenty minutes at a time.

So far, I've made sure to wear the dental device that helps my mandible return to normal placement after a night of wearing the Mandibular Advancement Device that treats my sleep apnea. I've also used the twenty minutes to peruse Twitter, email, and Facebook for kidney information via iPad. I've even done my banking online in this same twenty minutes.

As you can see, every minute of my time is important to me. That's why I was so glad to find new information that every minute you exercise counts. Obviously with my back sort-of- injury {I don't consider it an injury unless I can't walk!}, I've had to limit my exercise.

That's the bane of my existence anyway... not the limiting, but the exercise. I usually ride five or six miles on the stationary bike or do a two mile walking tape with weights and stretch bands. I have to admit, I do it only because I have to. I'd rather read or write anytime.

Although, I love my Sunday night exercise: the blues dance lesson my daughter, Abby, and her dance partner provide at The Blooze Bar. It's downright fun!

Back to every minute of exercise counts {Hurray!} This is the first paragraph of the news article about this study published on September 13th of this year. You can tell right away why I like it.

"A new study suggests something encouraging for busy people: Every minute of movement counts toward the 150 minutes of moderate-intensity physical activity we're all supposed to be getting each week. University of Utah researchers found that each minute spent engaging in some kind of moderate to vigorous physical activity was associated with lower BMI and lower weight."

I have to admit I don't break down that 150 minutes each week into daily totals when I think about exercise and it's overwhelming. Break it down and it's only a little less than 22 minutes a day. Hey, that's MY 22 minutes a day.

So what do they mean by "moderate-intensity physical exercise"?
I specifically looked at other than what we'd already consider
exercise which can be incorporated into your everyday activities.
I park a little further away from my destination than I need to whenever
I drive somewhere. If I'm not able to walk too well that day due to
plantar fasciitis, I'll chop vegetables or mix my from scratch pancake
batter by hand. If my hands hurt from arthritis or neuropathy that day,
I'll play with Bella – the cancer free wonder dog.

Wait a minute, these are all suggestions made in the study. And better yet, they count toward my 150 minutes of exercise a week. I like the idea that you don't have to chuck the whole idea of exercise if you don't have time to go to the gym, or climb your friendly, local mountain, or ride a bike 10 miles.

I especially like that my five minutes of rigorous dancing or riding the bike or exercising to those walking tapes count. Well, my five minutes usually turns into more since I figure I've started so I might as well finish my twenty minutes or thirty minutes of exercise that day.

Sunshine and Superwoman

10/20/14   Today is just one of those days: Bear's car is in the shop so I got up early to take him to work, I turned on the dishwasher and nothing happened, I posted what I thought was a non-political message and got a political rant in return, answered a text only to find that my childhood friend thought I was ignoring her. I've got a pretty happy life, so this was a disconcerting start of the day to say the least.

And then I opened the lab results for yet another blood test. The one I wrote about two weeks ago was from August; this one is from last week. Should have saved it for tomorrow.

While the out of range results weren't that much out of range, they were out of range. Since this is one of those days, all of a sudden this became of great concern to me.

The Vitamin D, 25-Hydroxy, Total was 28.6 instead of within the 30.1 - 100 normal range. It would probably help you understand my mystification if I let you know that I've been taking 2000 mg. of vitamin D daily for several years.

I went running right back to **What Is It and How Did I Get It? Early Stage Chronic Kidney Disease** to find out why this is important. Thank goodness, I have my office copy! How could anyone memorize everything they need to know about their health, I wonder. This is what I wrote about vitamin D {page 48}.

- The kidneys produce calcitrol which is the active form of vitamin D. The kidneys are the organs that transfer this vitamin from your food and skin [sunshine provides it to your skin] into something your body can use.
- Both vitamin D and calcium are needed for strong bones. It is yet another job of your kidneys to keep your bones strong and healthy.
- Should you have a deficit of Vitamin D, you'll need to be treated for this, in addition for any abnormal level of calcium or phosphates. The three work together.
- Vitamin D enables the calcium from the food you eat to be

> absorbed in the body. CKD may leech the calcium from your bones and body.
> - Phosphate levels can rise since this is stored in the blood and the bones as is calcium. With CKD, it's hard to keep the phosphate levels normal, so you may develop itchiness since the concentration of urea builds up and begins to crystallize through the skin. This is called pruritus.

I have been itchy lately, but since my phosphate levels have never been out of range, I concluded it was just dry skin due to our low to nil humidity here in Arizona. Maybe it's not. We'd been keeping my calcium levels low – but in range – since a bout with kidney stones several years ago. I also definitely stay out of the sun, another source of vitamin D, since a pre-cancerous face lesion. I'd had a bone density test recently and that was just fine, but had I been doing all the wrong things for my kidney health in protecting myself from kidney stones and melanoma?

Something was nagging at me about vitamin D, so I turned to the *Glossary* of my book {page 136} and that's where I found it:

Vitamin D: Regulates calcium and phosphorous blood levels as well as promoting bone formation, among other tasks – affects the immune system.

Affects the immune system. But how? Science Daily provided the answer I sought:

Scientists have found that vitamin D is crucial to activating our immune defenses and that without sufficient intake of the vitamin – the killer cells of the immune system — T cells — will not be able to react to and fight off serious infections in the body. The research team found that T cells first search for vitamin D in order to activate and if they cannot find enough of it will not complete the activation process.

How did I miss that? And how many others knew that vitamin D didn't just build strong bones as we'd been taught in primary school? I imagine my nephrologist will up my vitamin d dosage when I see him next week, but I still can't handle the sun or take calcium supplements. Maybe there's some food that can provide vast quantities of this vitamin.

But no, according to the National Institutes of Health:

Vitamin D is a fat-soluble vitamin that is naturally present in very few foods, added to others, and available as a dietary supplement.

Well, I wanted to know what those foods were even if they could only provide 20% of the needed vitamin D at most. I clearly remembered salmon, tuna, and egg yolks, but what else? Mushrooms, of course. And???

I had to turn to the internet for more suggestions. Fit Day informs us that milk, cereal, and even orange juice are vitamin d fortified. For me, that's a joke. I'm lactose intolerant, don't like cereal, and o.j. has too much calcium in it.

I like fish, but two to three times a week? I'm not sure I want to spend my five ounces of protein that way so often during a week. I don't care for eggs much, but am willing to eat them once a week just to eat something healthy. Mushrooms are really tasty, but my 1/4 cup daily doesn't go very far.

You know, just from moving myself to write, it doesn't seem like such a bad day after all.

Metabolic Syndrome doesn't Sit Well with Me

10/27/14   I have been dismayed by this spare tire around my middle for a while. I looked around and noticed some of my female friends have it, too. For some reason, I didn't look at my men friends' middles.

Was it a post-menopausal thing? No, not with these young women friends having it, too. So I asked and more than one told me she had Diabetes.

Whatever could that have to do with my spare tire, I wondered. I may be pre-diabetic, but I don't have diabetes. No, I think it's something else. So I researched and found I'd been in denial about having {self-diagnosed} Metabolic Syndrome. Certainly I'll speak with my primary care physician, but meanwhile I decided to tell you about it.

Did you know that one out of every three United States citizens and Canadian citizens suffer from Metabolic Syndrome? While the title sounds exotic, it's not. Okay, with those kinds of numbers, this isn't a case of Metabolic Syndrome being the disease – or syndrome – of the day. You know, when all of a sudden, everyone you know thinks {s}he has whatever it is… like me.

Okay, so what is it? This is what The Mayo Clinic had to say about it:

Metabolic syndrome is a cluster of conditions — increased blood pressure, a high blood sugar level, excess body fat around the waist and abnormal cholesterol levels — that occur together, increasing your risk of heart disease, stroke and diabetes.

Busted! On my August blood draw report, my blood sugar level was high at 6.2 via the A1C. That's what it's been for a year. Normal is between 4.8 and 5.6. A reading of 5.7 – 6.4 indicates increased risk for diabetes.

Just in case you don't remember, the Hemoglobin A1C measures how well your body handles blood sugar over a three month period. This is important for Chronic Kidney Disease patients because, as defined in ***What Is It and How Did I Get It? Early Stage Chronic Kidney Disease*** {page 132 for those with the book},

Hemoglobin: Transports oxygen in the blood via red blood cells and give the red blood cells their color.

Awk! I almost, but not quite, hesitated to check just how abnormal my cholesterol level was and for how long. I snuck a quite peek at my first book {page 130} before I did that just to be sure I knew what I was checking. The definition of cholesterol was:

While the basis for both sex hormones and bile, can cause blockages if it accumulated in the lining of a blood vessel.

So cholesterol is a good thing unless there's a buildup. Wait a minute; I need a refresher about bile. MedlinePlus cleared this up for me:

Bile is a fluid that is made and released by the liver and stored in the gallbladder. Bile helps with digestion. It breaks down fats into fatty acids, which can be taken into the body by the digestive tract.

My latest cholesterol reading {with medication to keep it low} for Total Cholesterol was in range {100 – 199} at 165, as was my HDL Cholesterol reading at 49 {Greater than 39 is acceptable}, my VLDL Cholesterol reading at 23 {5-40 is considered normal}, and my LDL Cholesterol reading {anywhere from 0 – 99 is normal}.

Let's backtrack just a bit. HDL is High Density Lipoprotein, the cholesterol that keeps your arteries clear or – as it's commonly called – the good cholesterol. VDL is Low Density Lipoprotein or the 'bad' kind that can clog your arteries. VLDL is Very Low Density Lipoprotein and one of the bad guys, too. It contains more triglycerides than protein and is big on clogging those arteries.

Hmmm, this is part of Metabolic Syndrome, but I didn't have it. Did I ever have a cholesterol problem? I looked back over the past year and noticed my Total Cholesterol had been out of whack by a point or two once or twice.

What about increased blood pressure? Well, I do have Chronic Kidney Disease and usually ran about 130/80. The 130 was the systolic part of the reading; it measured the pressure when the heart is beating. The lower part of the reading, or diastolic {The 80 in my case} was when the heart was at rest between beats. A normal blood pressure for a person my age {67} with CKD according to the new Eighth Joint National Committee is 150/90. Uh-oh, that's under control, too.

Having both your cholesterol and your blood pressure under control were good things, and in this case, they pointed out the folly of self-diagnose. Mea culpa!

By the way, this was important for CKD patients because we're already at risk for heart disease simply by being CKD patients. Why add to that risk with hypertension {high blood pressure} and/or hyperlipidemia {high cholesterol}?

Okay, so I didn't have Metabolic Syndrome despite the spare tire I carried. But maybe you do. Let's see what you can do about it. According to MedicineNet, the treatment is – you guessed it – diet, exercise, and no smoking. Medication is used if the syndrome is severe enough, but lifestyle changes are the first line of treatment.

Flanked by the Pain

11/3/14 The only thing consistent about this past week, like every week since I've been diagnosed with Chronic Kidney Disease is no kidney pain. Yet, a reader has told me she experiences pain in her kidneys although her doctors tell her this is not a symptom of kidney disease. Unfortunately, I neglected to ask what kind of kidney disease she has.

When I started researching, I found there are many different causes for kidney pain. MedicineNet informs us:

Some of the major underlying causes of kidney pain or flank pain are as follows:
- Urinary tract infections, mainly pyelonephritis
- Kidney stones
- Diabetes
- Glomerulonephritis
- High blood pressure
- Polycystic kidney disease (congenital)
- Congenital malformations in the renal system resulting in complete or partial blockage of urine flow
- Drugs or toxins that harm kidney tissue (for example, pesticide exposure or chronic use of medications such as ibuprofen [Advil, Motrin, and others])
- Drinking alcohol may cause acute or chronic flank pain; the pain source, depending on the individual, may be from the kidneys or the liver.

Wow! And doctors say kidney pain is not a symptom of CKD? Notice the two leading causes of CKD on this list: diabetes and high blood pressure. Oh, and the "drugs or toxins that harm kidney tissue…."

I clearly remember being asked if I had flank pain when I was first diagnosed… and I clearly remember asking where the flank was. For those of you, like me, who don't know, the primary definition of flank is:

the fleshy part of the side between the ribs and the hip.

Thank you for that, Merriam Webster Dictionary.

Then, never having experienced it myself, I had to know what it felt like – or at least find a description of the pain. eHealthStar {Which is a new site for me} describes it as:

- *Sudden (acute)* or *persistent (chronic)*
- *Mild* or *severe*
- *Sharp, dull, throbbing* or, rarely, *cramping or colicky*
- *One sided* or *both-sided.*

Kidney pain is often, but not always, associated with tenderness in the kidney area.

Wait a minute; that covers just about every kind of pain you can think of. So if you have a pain in your flank area, you have CKD – right? Wrong. Remember the list of other possible causes. We're familiar with kidney stones – a crystallization of mineral and acid salts that form a stone in the kidneys – which are not CKD. The 'C' in CKD is for chronic or long term, in this case long term deterioration of your kidney function. Drinking, while it may affect CKD, is not CKD. If you drink and experience flank pain, it does not mean you have CKD nor that you're going to develop CKD. Although, it might not be a bad idea to be tested should you have your suspicions. Speak to your primary care doctor about this. Numerous urinary tract infections may be a cause of CKD, but a single urinary tract infection may not. Even if you've had numerous UTIs, this does not mean that the pain from these indicates CKD.

Although…. Pyelonephritis, an infection of the kidneys is a more serious UTI as explained by WebMD:

Most cases of pyelonephritis are complications of common bladder infections. Bacteria enter the body from the skin around the urethra. They then travel up the urethra to the bladder. Sometimes, bacteria escape the bladder and urethra, traveling up the ureters to one or both kidneys.

Pyelonephritis is a potentially serious kidney infection that can spread to the blood, causing severe illness. Fortunately, pyelonephritis is almost always curable with antibiotics.

This makes quite a bit of sense. The second nephrologist to treat me referred me to an urologist when he realized I was on my fifth UTI in the same summer and he suspected this one had spread to my bladder. The urologist actually had me look through the cystoscope myself to reassure me that the lower urinary tract infection had not spread to the upper urinary tract where the bladder is located. Believe me, it felt surreal to be able to look inside my own body in real time.

Notice I'm exploring all the items on the list although not in the order MedicineNet.com offers them. What's next?

Let's take a look at Glomerulonephritis. I went right back to my old friend The Mayo Clinic for some answers. That's where I found this definition of the disease.

Glomerulonephritis (gloe-mer-u-low-nuh-FRY-tis) is inflammation of the tiny filters in your kidneys (glomeruli). Glomeruli remove excess fluid, electrolytes and waste from your bloodstream and pass them into your urine. Also called glomerular disease, glomerulonephritis can be acute — a sudden attack of inflammation — or chronic — coming on gradually.

So this one does have more to do with the kidneys, but it's still not CKD. It can be acute, which Chronic Kidney Disease cannot. Obviously, congenital diseases or malfunctions of the kidney are also not CKD since you are born with them, rather than having a slow deterioration of your kidney function.

For the life of me {Cute, huh?}, I cannot understand why a nephrologist would tell a CKD patient that flank – or kidney – pain cannot be associated with CKD when this may be one of the symptoms. I'm going to have to suggest to the reader that asked for this blog that she challenge her nephrologist... again.

Pro on Probiotics?

11/10/14 My husband takes probiotics and they work for him. This is why he takes them, as explained by Theralac.

For healthy people, probiotics can help boost the immune system and increase the absorption of important minerals and nutrients. For people with digestive problems, probiotics can be taken in higher doses to help regain digestive balance.

I thought they might be worth a try, but my nephrologist disagreed. We had our discussion about this right after I'd been a guest on a radio show during which the pros and cons of using probiotics for Chronic Kidney Disease were discussed. This was just about the same time the information I'd requested from Kibow arrived. This is from their website:

Certain probiotic microorganisms can utilize urea, uric acid and creatinine and other toxins as its nutrients for growth. Overloaded and impaired kidneys have a buildup of these poisonous wastes in the bloodstream. Probiotic microorganisms multiply, thereby creating a greater diffusion of these uremic toxins from the circulating blood across the lining of the intestinal walls into the bowel. This increased microbial growth is excreted along with the feces (which is normally 50% microbes by weight).

Enteric toxin reduction technology uses probiotic organisms to transform the colon into a blood cleansing agent, which, with the aid of microbes, indirectly removes toxic wastes and helps eliminate them as fecal matter. Consequently, a natural treatment for kidney failure is possible to maintain a healthy kidney function with the oral use of Renadyl™. The patented, proprietary probiotics in Renadyl™ have been clinically tested and shown to be safe, free of serious side effects, and effective in helping the body rid itself of harmful toxins when taken for as long as 6 months.

Let's slow down a bit. We'll need some definitions, so I turned to my favorite user friendly Merriam-Webster online medical dictionary for the following.

CREATININE: {I know you know this one; this is just a reminder} a white crystalline strongly basic compound $C_4H_7N_3O$ formed from creatine and found especially in muscle, blood, and urine

ENTERIC: of, relating to or affecting the intestines; *broadly*: alimentary

PROBIOTIC: a preparation (as a dietary supplement) containing a live bacterium (as lactobacilli) that is taken orally to restore beneficial bacteria to the body; *also*: a bacterium of such a preparation

UREA: a substance that contains nitrogen, is found in the urine of mammals and some fish, and is used in some kinds of fertilizer

URIC ACID: a white odorless and tasteless nearly insoluble acid $C_5H_4N_4O_3$ that is the chief nitrogenous waste present in the urine especially of lower vertebrates (as birds and reptiles), is present in small quantity in human urine, and occurs pathologically in renal calculi {A little help here: this means a concretion usually of mineral salts around organic material found especially in hollow organs or ducts} and the tophi of gout

What I found on Kibow is a mouthful… and an advertisement. I am not endorsing Renadyl. I'm still leery of that six month warning, especially after I found the following at the bottom of one of their pages:

* These statements have not been approved by the Food and Drug Administration. This product is not intended to diagnose, treat, cure or prevent disease. Results may vary.

In addition, this product contains psyllium seed husk, something I was cautioned to avoid. It seems my nephrologist is not the only one who feels this way. Metamucil, a product whose main ingredient is psyllium, is a conscientious company that also posts this information on their website.

Psyllium Products and Their Minerals

There are certain psyllium products that contain a large amount of minerals that individuals with kidney disease cannot process. Some psyllium products contain high volumes of potassium, sodium and magnesium, which if a person with kidney disease consumes can cause a lot of problems. If an individual's physician gives permission on taking psyllium then they need to make sure the psyllium product follows their restricted diet.

Fluids Required With Psyllium
When consuming psyllium six to eight glasses of water must be consumed to keep from having any uncomfortable side effects. This can be a problem for an individual with kidney disease since the kidneys cannot effectively filter the fluid. Since the proper amount of fluid cannot be consumed this can cause side effects and make the natural fiber less effective.

Things to Consider
One of the number one complaints in individuals with kidney disease is constipation due to the fact fluid restrictions, vegetables and more. Since there are many restrictions an individual has with kidney disease with their diet there are other safe options to choose from. Discuss these other safe options with your physician to relieve constipation.

Maybe it's just me, but I don't understand why someone with kidney disease would want to take a product that will harm them. As a matter of fact, I don't understand why Kibow, the makers of Renadyl, don't post such a warning on their site. Hmmm, I wonder if the "...safe, free of serious side effects, and effective in helping the body rid itself of harmful toxins when taken for as long as 6 months" statement included in their material IS their warning. And just how many people catch that one sentence anyway?

I did find the record of a study filed by Kibow in 2009, but not the results of the six month trial. The record was processed on November 9, 2014 which is very recent. Either I don't know how to find the outcomes of the trial or they are simply not there. I suspect the latter.

I have no intention of vilifying Kibow, but do find this to be another case of be careful what you choose to take, very careful. Watch the small print, talk to your nephrologist before making any decisions, and make sure you guard whatever you have left of your kidney function.

Up and Down...and Up...and Down

11/17/14   There's been some variation in my eGFR for the last few months and it hasn't all been good. What's the eGFR, you ask. Let's start with the GFR and use the *Glossary* in ***What Is It and How Did I Get It? Early Stage Chronic Kidney Disease*** {page 132} for the definition.

Glomerular filtration rate [if there is a lower case "e" before the term, it means estimated glomerular filtration rate] which determines both the stage of kidney disease and how well the kidneys are functioning.

Wonderful, except we need to know what glomerulus means since the suffix 'ar' tells us that glomerular is an adjective or word that describes a noun – a person, place, thing, or idea. In this case, the noun is glomerulus.   Thank you, dictionary.reference.com for the following:

Also called Malpighian tuft, a tuft of convoluted capillaries in the nephron of a kidney, functioning to remove certain substances from the blood before it flows into the convoluted tubule.

Yes, yes, I know more definitions are needed. Back to the *Glossary* in ***What Is It and How Did I Get It? Early Stage Chronic Kidney Disease*** {page 134 this time}

Nephrons: The part of the kidney that actually purifies and filters the blood.

A tubule, as you've probably guessed, is a very small tube. This is when having been an English teacher for decades pays off in my kidney work! Maybe we should define capillary too, in case you've forgotten what it is. This time I used Merriam-Webster.com at MedlinePlus:

a minute thin-walled vessel of the body; especially: any of the smallest blood vessels connecting arteriole with venules and forming networks throughout the body.

In other words, they're the smallest blood vessels in the body.

Alright, we've got our vocabulary in place; now why is the eGFR so important? As stated in the definition above, it is used for staging your Chronic Kidney Disease. Different stages require different treatment or no treatment at all. There are five stages with the mid-level stage divided into two parts. The higher the stage, the worse your kidney function.

Think of the stages as a test with 100 being the highest score. These are the stages and their treatments.

STAGE 1: (normal or high) – above 90 – usually requires watching, not treatment, although many people decide to make life style changes now: following a renal diet, exercising, lowering blood pressure, ceasing to smoke, etc.

STAGE 2: (mild) - 60-89 – Same as for stage one

STAGE 3A: (moderate) - 45-59 – This is when you are usually referred to a nephrologist {kidney specialist}. You'll need a renal {kidney} dietitian, too, since you need to be rigorous in avoiding more than certain amounts of protein, potassium, phosphorous, and sodium in your diet to slow down the deterioration of your kidneys. Each patient has different needs so there is no one diet. The diet is based on your lab results. Medications such as those for high blood pressure may be prescribed to help preserve your kidney function.

STAGE 3B: (moderate) - 30-44 – same as above, except the patient may experience symptoms.

STAGE 4: (severe 15-29) – Here's when dialysis may start. A kidney transplant may be necessary instead of dialysis {artificial cleansing of your blood}. Your nephrologist will probably want to see you every three months and request labs before each visit.

STAGE 5: (End stage) - below 15 – Dialysis or transplant is necessary to continue living.

Many thanks to DaVita for refreshing my memory about each stage.

Back to my original concern about the GFR results in my labs. Why did it fluctuate from 53 in August of last year, to 47 in February of this year, to

52 in May, to 56 in August, and to 47 last week? All the values are within stage 3A and I know it's only a total fluctuation of six points, but it's my fluctuation so I want to know. And that's what started this whole blog about GFR.

I discovered that different labs may use slightly different calculations to estimate your GFR, but I always go to the same lab, the one in my doctor's office. Nope, that's not my answer.

According to the American Kidney Fund:

...this test may not be accurate if you are younger than 18, pregnant, very overweight or very muscular.

No, these situations don't apply to me either. Maybe I'm going about this all wrong and should look at the formula for arriving at GFR. The National Kidney Disease Education program lists the formula which includes your serum creatinine. Aha! Maybe that's the cause of the variation.

First a reminder: creatinine is the chemical waste product of muscle use. {This is a highly simplified definition.} You'll find this on your Comprehensive Metabolic Panel Blood Results, should you have your results. The normal values are between 0.57 and 1.00 mg/dL. Mine were above normal for each test, a sign that I have CKD. As if I didn't already know that. These results were also lower each time my GFR was higher.

I researched and researched. My final understanding is that not only can CKD elevate your creatinine, but so can dehydration, diabetes or high blood pressure. If your creatinine is elevated, the results of the GFR formula will be lowered. That's enough information to allow me to rest easy until I see my doctor next week.

Some of this was pretty technical, but you may want to try an online GFR calculator just to see how it works. You will need your serum creatinine value {Serum means blood, so this is not to be confused with the urine creatinine test} to do so. I like the one at DaVita.

Smokin'!

11/24/13   When I was in college a million years ago, this was a compliment. I'd wear the new dress my mother bought me, go to a dance or a party, dance my brains out, and find some guys whispering this under their breath as I passed them.

Not anymore. True, Mom's long gone, I'm married, and if anyone whispered this to me now, I'd think they were asking me if I smoked...and that's a big no-no these days, especially with Chronic Kidney Disease.

We've taken for granted for years now that people just don't smoke anymore. That's not true, you know. Other countries still find smoking acceptable, although not all. There are also people who are so addicted that they just can't stop. Today we'll take a look at what might help.

But first, we need to go back to the basics – as usual. On my very first visit to a nephrologist, I was told to stop smoking, even social smoking. But why? DaVita offered a succinct answer to my question.

How smoking can harm kidneys
- Increases blood pressure and heart rate
- Reduces blood flow in the kidneys
- Increases production of angiotensin II (a hormone produced in kidney)
- Narrows the blood vessels in the kidneys
- Damages arterioles (branches of arteries)
- Forms arteriosclerosis (thickening and hardening) of the renal arteries
- Accelerates loss of kidney function

In addition to tobacco, smoking allows other toxins into the body. And according to the American Association of Kidney Patients (AAKP), studies have shown that smoking is harmful for the kidneys, and can cause kidney disease to progress and increases the risk for proteinuria {Excessive amount of protein in the urine}.

To make this a little more comprehensive, here are some definitions from ***What Is It and How Did I Get It? Early Stage Chronic Kidney Disease.***

Arteries: Vessels that carry blood *from* the heart.

Hormones: …chemicals that trigger tissues to do whatever their particular job is.

Protein: Amino acids arranged in chains joined by peptide bonds to form a compound, important because some proteins are hormones, enzymes, and antibodies.

Renal: Of or about the kidneys

Sounds drastic, doesn't it? So, what can be done to help those people who are so addicted they can't stop smoking on their own?

An Israeli PhD student at Weizmann Institute of Science in Rehovot, Anat Arzi, has a novel idea. She believes that exposing smokers to the smell of smoke and other unpleasant odors while they sleep can make them less eager to smoke. In her own words:

This research stems from recent findings suggesting that novel associations can be learned during human sleep and retrieved upon awakening.

While this was only a small study with 76 people, I can't remember reading about any other cease smoking study that deals with aversive conditioning during REM sleep. Aversive conditioning is just what it sounds like: using unpleasant stimuli – like the rotten fish Arzi used – to cause some kind of change in behavior. Quick reminder, REM means Rapid Eye Movement and occurs during the second stage of falling asleep.

Then, there's the FDA approved, safe, natural product Smoke Remedy offered on the internet. You need to remember that FDA approved, safe, and natural does not necessarily mean safe for CKD. I applaud the fact that they list their ingredients, but this is not safe for us.
The homeopathic medicines in Smoke Remedy™ come from several

different plant and mineral sources that include:

- Avena sativa – to help with the addiction to nicotine and tobacco;
- Caladium seguinum, Daphne Indica, Eugenia jambosa, Ignatia, Calcarea phosphorica, and Plantago major – these help to stop the craving and desire to smoke;
- Kali phosphoricum, Nux vomica, and Staphysagria – to help prevent the withdrawal symptoms you may experience when quitting;
- The product also contains purified water, citric acid and potassium sorbate.

For example, that last ingredient, potassium sorbate caught my eye because we know that we, as people with CKD, need to limit our potassium. It turns out to be a preservative and nothing I'd want in my body whether the FDA approves it or not. The Calcarea Phosphorica made me pause, too. As CKD patients, we do not need more phosphorous, as you already know.

I'm not saying don't use homeopathic remedies, but I am saying you need to research each and every ingredient AND bring the list of side effects to your nephrologist before you do. Your doctor may not be familiar with homeopathic medicines, which is why you are doing the research to bring to him or her.

Of course, there's always the patch or special gums, but they have their own problems. Most feed slow doses of nicotine into your body. That's the element of tobacco that injures your kidneys. This is to address the withdrawal symptoms.

I went to StopSmoking.net to see if there are side effects. Don't you just love products with full disclosure? Here's what I found:

It's worth noting that many of the top nicotine patches often produce undesirable side effects. Common side effects include headaches, dizziness, upset stomach, nausea, chest pain, breathing problems, anxiety, and irregular heartbeat. Furthermore, some people have nicotine patch allergies. The skin becomes red, and their body becomes severely irritated by the patch. If this ever happens, you need to contact a doctor right away. Nicotine patch allergies can produce damaging results.

Now here's an eye opener I found at The Chart.

"The perception of the public using the product is that these are good forever – that these will result in you not smoking in three, five, 10 years," says Greg Connolly, Director of the Center for Global Tobacco Control at the Harvard School of Public Health. "Well, they were never designed to do that. They were designed to treat withdrawal, which is a symptom that occurs from stopping to probably six months, and then it usually ends."

I never realized how really hard it is for addicted smokers to stop. Now I fully appreciate my father who decided there wasn't enough money coming in for him to waste it on cigarettes when he had three children. He simply stopped. Or so I thought. {This was way before 1996 when the patch and gum first made their appearance.} Thank you, Dad; this must have been really hard.

She's Got Good Bones… or Does She?

12/1/14   Thanksgiving was wonderful, just plain wonderful. I'm lucky. All the kids know about my Chronic Kidney Disease and accept my limitations. There's no exclaiming that I must have a glass of the family's favorite Moscato or eat some of the Hungarian Strudel our host baked. I didn't even mind cooking the sweet potato-pineapple-marshmallow dish I wasn't going to eat or smelling the delicious aroma of the string bean casserole with cream of mushroom soup and fried onions atop it Bear prepared that I knew I also wasn't going to eat. I had what I wanted: almost all the kids together under one roof with Bear and me. Food was secondary.

How do I go from Thanksgiving dinner to the osteoporosis a reader asked me to write about? Ah, I know. Food contains vitamins, right? One of the causes of this bone disease is a vitamin D deficiency. How many of you are taking vitamin D supplements? Raise your hands. Wow, that's everyone in the room {I am raising my hand as I sit alone in my office writing this blog}. And what does this vitamin D insufficiency have to do with your Chronic Kidney Disease? Does anyone remember?

Ah, great idea! Let's go back to **What Is It and How Did I Get It? Early Stage Chronic Kidney Disease** for the answer. That is on page 48 or you can use a phrase search for the digital version.

- The kidneys produce calcitrol which is the active form of vitamin D. The kidneys are the organs that transfer this vitamin from your food and skin [sunshine provides it to your skin] into something your body can use.
- Both vitamin D and calcium are needed for strong bones. It is yet another job of your kidneys to keep your bones strong and healthy.
- Should you have a deficit of Vitamin D, you'll need to be treated for this, in addition for any abnormal level of calcium or phosphates. The three work together.
- Vitamin D enables the calcium from the food you eat to be absorbed in the body. CKD may leech the calcium from your bones and body.

- Phosphate levels can rise since this is stored in the blood and the bones as is calcium. With CKD, it's hard to keep the phosphate levels normal, so you may develop itchiness since the concentration of urea builds up and begins to crystallize through the skin. This is called pruritus.

Did you catch that fourth point – leeching? So now we know how the lack of vitamin D, common in Chronic Kidney Disease patients, can be a factor in having osteoporosis, but what is osteoporosis? According to The National Osteoporosis Foundation:

Osteoporosis means "porous bone." If you look at healthy bone under a microscope, you will see that parts of it look like a honeycomb. If you have osteoporosis, the holes and spaces in the honeycomb are much bigger than they are in healthy bone. This means your bones have lost density or mass and that the structure of your bone tissue has become abnormal. As your bones become less dense, they also become weaker and more likely to break. If you're age 50 or older and have broken a bone, talk to your doctor or other healthcare provider and ask if you should have a bone density test.

Both Bear and I have had this test since we are both over 50 and have broken bones, several for each of us in fact. I am pleased to announce that neither one of us has a bone density problem. The test itself was simple. Here's an explanation of what it entails from The Mayo Clinic:

If you have your bone density test done at a hospital, it'll probably be done on a central device, where you lie on a padded platform while a mechanical arm passes over your body. The amount of radiation you're exposed to is very low, much less than the amount emitted during a chest X-ray. The test usually takes about 10 to 30 minutes.

A small, portable machine can measure bone density in the bones at the far ends of your skeleton, such as those in your finger, wrist or heel. The instruments used for these tests are called peripheral devices, and are often found in pharmacies. Tests of peripheral bone density are considerably less expensive than are tests done on central devices.

Because bone density can vary from one location in your body to another, a measurement taken at your heel usually isn't as accurate a predictor of fracture risk as is a measurement taken at your spine or hip. That's why, if your test on a peripheral device is positive, your doctor might recommend a follow-up scan at your spine or hip to confirm your diagnosis.

Unfortunately, osteoporosis is common with CKD. That word is common, not universal. While you may want to be careful about your vitamin D levels to make certain you have enough, there's no reason to be unduly alarmed. We have Chronic Kidney Disease. Our systems are already compromised. This is only one of the POSSIBLE risks of our disease.

Faster! Faster! The Holidays are Coming

12/8/14 Too often, we're tempted to grab something fast along the way. You and I, my friends, cannot do that as Chronic Kidney Disease sufferers. It turns out our friends and families really can't either.

Healthline.com kindly sent this to me just at the right time. I'll let them present their case and comment throughout. Due to space constraints, I've omitted the portions that pertain to children. You can read those and take a look at the infograph for this information on Healthline's website.

Effects of Fast Food on the Body
Food is fuel for your body and has a direct impact on how you feel as well as on your overall health. Fast food refers to food that can be served quickly. In many cases, that means food that is highly processed and contains large amounts of carbohydrates, added sugar, unhealthy fats, and salt (sodium). These foods generally contain a high number of calories but offer little or no nutritional value. {Oh no, not sodium.}

Eating out added between 160 and 310 extra calories a day. According to the National Institutes of Health, some fast food meals give you a whole day's worth of calories. That can really pack on the pounds. Being overweight is a risk factor for a variety of chronic health problems.)like the obesity which may lead to diabetes, which just happens to be the leading cause of Chronic Kidney Disease.} When fast food frequently replaces nutritious foods in your diet, it can lead to poor nutrition and poor health.

Digestive and Cardiovascular Systems
Many fast foods and drinks are loaded with carbohydrates and, consequently, a lot of calories. Your digestive system breaks carbs down into sugar (glucose), which it then releases into your bloodstream. Your pancreas responds by releasing insulin, which is needed to transport sugar to cells throughout your body. As the sugar is absorbed, your blood sugar levels drop. When blood sugar gets low, your pancreas releases another hormone called glucagon. Glucagon tells the liver to start making use of stored sugars. When everything is working in sync, blood sugar levels stay within a normal range.

When you take in high amounts of carbs, it causes a spike in your blood sugar. That can alter the normal insulin response. Frequent spikes in blood sugar may be a contributing factor in insulin resistance and type 2 diabetes. {Is anyone else pre-diabetic like me?}

Added sugars have no nutritional value but are high in calories. According to the American Heart Association, most Americans take in twice as many sugars as is recommended for optimal health. All those extra calories add up to extra weight, a contributing factor in heart disease.

Trans fats, often found in fast food, are known to raise LDL cholesterol levels. That's the undesirable kind of cholesterol. It can also lower HDL cholesterol. That's the good cholesterol. Trans fats may also increase your risk of developing type 2 diabetes.

Too much sodium helps to retain water, so it can cause general bloating and puffiness. Sodium can contribute to high blood pressure {which, as we know, is the second leading cause of CKD} or enlarged heart muscle. If you have congestive heart failure, cirrhosis, or **KIDNEY DISEASE** {my bolding and capitalization in this paragraph.}, too much salt can contribute to a dangerous build-up of fluid. Excess sodium may also increase risk for kidney stones, **KIDNEY DISEASE**, and stomach cancer. High cholesterol and high blood pressure are among the top risk factors for heart disease and stroke.

Respiratory System
Obesity is associated with an increase in respiratory problems, and treating those ailments may be more complicated. Even without diagnosed medical conditions, obesity may cause episodes of shortness of breath or wheezing with little exertion. Obesity may play a role in the development of sleep apnea {Read the blog about how this affects CKD.} and asthma.

Central Nervous System
There are many types of headache and many things that can cause them. Some dietary triggers that can be found in fast food include salt, processed meats, nitrates, and MSG.

A study published in the journal Public Health Nutrition showed that eating commercial baked goods (doughnuts, croissants, cake) and fast food (pizza, hamburgers, hot dogs) {Does this remind you of your renal diet?} may be linked to depression. People who eat fast food are 51 percent more likely to develop depression than those who eat little to no fast food. It was also found that the more fast food they consumed, the more likely study participants were to develop depression.

Skin and Bones
Chocolate and greasy foods, often blamed for acne, are not the real culprits. It's carbs. According to The Mayo Clinic, because foods that are high in carbohydrates increase blood sugar levels, they may also trigger acne.

When you consume foods high in carbs and sugar, bacteria residing in your mouth produce acids. Those acids are hard on your teeth. In fact, they can destroy tooth enamel, a contributing factor in dental cavities. When the enamel of your tooth is lost, it can't be replaced. Poor oral health has also been linked to other health problems. {Maybe it's time for another blog on CKD and your teeth.}

Excess sodium may also increase your risk of developing osteoporosis (thin, fragile bones). {My, my, how interconnected it all is. CKD affects your bones, too.}

Many thanks to Maggie Danhakl, Assistant Marketing Manager at Healthline, for making sure this showed up in my mailbox exactly when we needed it.

Renal Arterial Stenosis, Huh?

12/15/14 I recently attended a social function at which someone I respect tapped me on the shoulder and said, "Make sure you speak with our mutual friend before you leave." So I did … and was mystified when she conducted some small talk with me. This is what he wanted me to hear?

Later I received a message from our mutual friend and all became clear. She'd been diagnosed with renal arterial stenosis and her doctor wanted her to have surgery. Could I help? At that point, I couldn't, but I could research for her and I did.

Then I got to thinking about how many of us with Chronic Kidney Disease don't know what this is or what it might have to do with us, other than it starts with renal – which is from the Latin for kidneys. The Greek root is 'neph' as in nephrology.

I turned to **What Is It and How Did I Get It? Early Stage Chronic Kidney Disease** {page 129} for the definition of arteries:

Vessels that carry blood *from* the heart.

So, we're looking at vessels attached to the kidneys that bring in blood from the heart. And why do we need that I wondered? Oh wait. I remember: the kidneys filter this blood and then send it back to your heart via the veins. That's where stenosis comes in. According to the medical dictionary, this is:

a constriction or narrowing of a duct or passage; a stricture.

That same dictionary gave us a precise definition of renal artery stenosis:

narrowing of one or both renal arteries, so that renal function is impaired, resulting in renal hypertension and, if stenosis is bilateral, chronic renal failure

So what we're looking at here is a narrowing of the artery that brings blood from the heart to the kidneys for cleaning by the nephrons.

Now hold on there. Let's not panic, folks. This does not mean automatic chronic renal failure and dialysis or transplant.

Let's take a look at what might cause renal artery stenosis or RAS. I went directly to a trusted site, U.S. Department of Health And Human Services, National Kidney and Urologic Diseases Information Clearinghouse (NKUDIC), A service of the National Institute of Diabetes and Digestive and Kidney Diseases (NIDDK).

About 90 percent of RAS is caused by atherosclerosis—clogging, narrowing, and hardening of the renal arteries. In these cases, RAS develops when plaque - a sticky substance made up of fat, cholesterol, calcium, and other material found in the blood - builds up on the inner wall of one or both renal arteries. Plaque buildup is what makes the artery wall hard and narrow.

Most other cases of RAS are caused by fibromuscular dysplasia (FMD)— the abnormal development or growth of cells on the renal artery walls— which can cause blood vessels to narrow. Rarely, RAS is caused by other conditions.

Our mutual friend had been making herself out to be a terrible person to herself, one who caused her own RAS. Well, maybe she did... and maybe she didn't. It could have been FMD or some other unknown condition. If it wasn't, I still can't see her blaming herself if she didn't know about preventing atherosclerosis. The point is she does now and needs to deal with the RAS.

MedicineNet tells us that symptoms aren't that common.

In general, renal artery stenosis is not associated with any obvious or specific symptoms. Suspicious signs for renal artery stenosis include:
- high blood pressure that responds poorly to treatment;
- severe high blood pressure that develops prior to age 30 or greater than age 50;
- an incidental finding (discovered through routine tests or tests performed for another condition) of one small kidney compared to a normal sized one on the other side.

Typically, unilateral (one-sided) renal artery stenosis may be related to high blood pressure whereas bilateral (two-sided) renal artery stenosis is more often related to diminished kidney function.

What about that surgery our mutual friend's doctor wanted her to have? Is it really necessary?

Sometimes a regiment of several hypertension {high blood pressure} drugs, along with hyperlipidemia {high cholesterol} drugs, and perhaps aspirin can alleviate the problem. Then there's angioplasty – a procedure in which a catheter is placed in the artery via a blood vessel, a balloon is then opened in the artery and stented to keep the renal artery open. Or, bypass surgery may be performed to avoid the blocked area of the renal artery. Thank you to WebMD for this information which I paraphrased.

My advice when surgery is suggested? A second opinion. Any doctor worth his salt will welcome this request and understand that it in no way casts aspersion on his/her value as a doctor. A second opinion from a nephrologist would be the way that I would go and I urged our mutual friend to seek one.

Here's to our mutual friend and all of us who ever wondered what RAS is and what it has to do with CKD.

On another note entirely, here's a bit of happiness I wanted to share with you. These are reviews for ***What Is It and How Did I Get It? Early Stage Chronic Kidney Disease*** I hadn't seen on Amazon.com... and all five stars!
- One of the best on the subject not so much for the info but the way it was presented. Almost like a novel. Makes you forget your kidney is not behaving the way it should.
- It is written for a patient like us, mean that the language it is simple and easy to understand, good sense of humor and a positive aptitude with this silent killer, another book that deserve a place on your personal library. Very informative, excellent book.
- A book that is very helpful to CKD3 patients. It gives the facts and figures needed most to those with this condition!

- I've had this book in paperback for a while and when Amazon offered me the option to buy the digital version at a discounted price since I had purchased the paperback from them, I jumped at it. I'm a sucker for loaning out hard copy and this way if I find a fellow kidney disease sufferer, I can let them have my paperback and I will always have my digital backup for reference. This is a great book by a fellow kidney disease patient who also publishes a very good blog. There are so many details to track with this disease and she talks about the daily life of it. Very helpful and answers so many questions. She's a born researcher, so all her information has backup links to let you know this is authentic medical advice to get some of those questions answered between doctor's visits.

It's Different

12/22/14 Sometime ago, I mentioned that Dr. Andrew Weill was my health guru. I felt that way after my now deceased best buddy introduced me to the wonders of healthy eating. I miss her… and him.

Why him? As you know a healthy diet is not a renal healthy diet. I still subscribe to his Nutrition Newsletter. Today, vegetables and fruits were discussed including some excellent advice, but not specifically for us as Chronic Kidney Disease patients.

Colorizing Your Diet

Phytonutrients - the chemical compounds in plants that appear to protect health, but are not established as essential nutrients - are generally concentrated in the skins of many vegetables and fruits, and are responsible for their vibrant hues, scents and flavors. Some phytonutrients are powerful anti-inflammatory agents; others modulate and enhance immune function, maintaining the body's healing system while keeping abnormal inflammation in check; and still others boost antioxidant defenses to protect DNA and other cellular components from toxic insults that can cause direct harm, or can promote abnormal inflammation leading to tissue damage.

In order to get the full range of protective phytonutrients, you should "colorize" your diet: include fresh produce from all parts of the color spectrum and aim for one serving per day (one-half cup cooked or one cup raw) of a fruit or vegetable from all the various color groups (red, red-purple, orange, orange-yellow, yellow-green, green and white-green).

Okay, we're pretty sure CKD is an inflammatory disease so this would make sense. We already have compromised systems, so we can use that immune function enhancement. And we certainly won't say no to something that can protect our cells and DNA from toxic insults. So what's the problem?

Let me answer it this way. In *Chapter 8: The Renal Diet* of **What Is It and How Did I Get It? Early Stage Chronic Kidney Disease** on page 73, I wrote the following.

In order to fully understand the renal diet, you need to know a little something about electrolytes. There are the sodium, potassium, and phosphate you've been told about and also calcium, magnesium, chloride and bicarbonate. They maintain balance in your body. This is not the kind of balance that helps you stand upright, but the kind that keeps your body healthy. Too much or too little of a certain electrolyte presents different problems. Eating a larger portion than suggested in the renal diet of a low sodium, phosphate, protein or potassium food is the equivalent of eating a high sodium, phosphate, protein or potassium food.

So it's not just eating the fruits and vegetables from each color group. We need to analyze the electrolytes in each serving, especially the phosphate and potassium. I also can only eat three servings of fruits and three of vegetables rather than the seven Dr. Weil recommends.

Why the restrictions of the electrolytes?

Let's take a look at potassium. Potassium is not a bad thing if you don't have CKD. It dumps wastes from your cells and helps the kidneys, heart and muscles to function normally. However, too much can cause irregular heartbeat and even heart attacks. Your kidneys are not doing an effective job of filtering the potassium in your blood. You have CKD. This should explain the connection between CKD and cardiovascular events.

And phosphorous? I'll quote from **What Is It and How Did I Get It? Early Stage Chronic Kidney Disease** again here since I like the simple direct way I explained it on page 76.

This is the second most plentiful mineral in the body and works closely with the first, calcium. Together, they produce strong bones and teeth. 85% of the phosphorous and calcium in our bodies is stored in the bones and teeth. The rest circulates in the blood except for about 5% that is in cells and tissues. Again, phosphorous is important for the kidneys since it filters out waste via them. Phosphorous balances and metabolizes other vitamins and minerals including vitamin D which is so important to CKD patients. As usual, it performs other functions, such as getting oxygen to tissues and changing protein, fat and carbohydrate into energy.

Be aware that kidney disease can cause excessive phosphorus. And what does that mean for Early Stage CKD patients? Not much if the phosphorous levels are kept low. Later, at Stages 4 and 5, bone problems including pain and breakage may be endured since excess phosphorous means the body tries to maintain balance by using the calcium that should be going to the bones. There are other consequences, but this is the one most easily understood.

To complicate matters even more, CKD patients are limited to different servings sizes of different fruits and vegetables, not the straight across the board ½ cup cooked or 1 cup raw of each Dr. Weil suggests. For example: I can eat ½ cup of broccoli, but only 1/3 cup of raisins. It depends upon the electrolytes in the particular fruit and vegetable and how much of that specific electrolyte you've eaten that day. *sigh* I miss the days of having Dr. Weil as my health guru.

I found even more reviews and all five stars! I am so enjoying this. Thank you all for the reviews.

- I was just diagnosed with Chronic Kidney disease Stage 4 a few weeks ago and I want to THANK YOU very much for this book. I put it on my Kindle. It is written in a way that one newly diagnosed and not in the medical field can understand.
- Gail Rae has provided a good insight to the bombshell that befalls millions of unsuspecting humans worldwide. A CKD victim myself with years of experience under my belt, found the book extremely informative and a great reference when providing peer support to newly diagnosed sufferers of this silent killer.
- So much good information for Chronic Kidney Disease Patients, from beginning to end. Thank you Gail Rae.
- Ms. Rae knows, in my opinion, what she is talking about. She is direct-to the point-and the book is easily understood. She has just a hint of humor in her writing which keeps the reader engaged. Will keep this in my reference library.

Auld Lang … Ah Choo!

12/29/14 Happy middle of Kwanzaa. I hope your Chanukah, Christmas, or whatever else you may celebrate that I don't know about was merry, too. Ours was…maybe even too merry. Even with cutting out overt sugar and dairy and sticking to the renal diet, I felt like I was getting sick. Too much running around? The stress of this happy season? Who knows, but there it was.

One of my daughters heard it in my voice and asked me why I just didn't take Airborne and nip whatever this was in the bud. I knew I couldn't, but I'd forgotten why. Hello, today's blog. This is not a blog to vilify this product, but one to inform you why we – as Chronic Kidney Disease patients – cannot take any product of this ilk.

Let's start at the beginning. According to their website, this is the short list of what's in Airborne.

Vitamins and Minerals
• Vitamin C: Antioxidants that go to work on the cellular level to quench free radicals and support cellular health. Vitamin C also supports the function of immune cells throughout your body.
• Vitamin E: Naturally-occurring antioxidant nutrients that inactivate harmful free radicals
• Vitamin A: Phyto-nutrients that work as antioxidants, on the cellular level, to promote immunity and protect DNA
• Zinc: An essential nutrient that works as a trigger for over 200 different enzymes and supports the number and function of several different immune cells.
• Selenium, Manganese, Magnesium: All minerals that support immunity

Okay, so what is the problem here? I needed more information since their website called this the "short list," so I marched into my pharmacy, took a look at the ingredients, and physically backed up.

I already knew that Vitamin C could promote kidney stones and that I was prone to those, having already had one. Wait a minute. 1633% of the daily value? We all know I'm not a doctor, but that sounds like asking for a kidney stone to me.

This is not to say you need to completely avoid Vitamin C. You need it; just not in such high doses. The per cent I quoted above is for one dose, but the instructions for Airborne direct you take this up to three times a day. In other words, triple that percentage.

Backtrack time. This is why you need this particular vitamin. Vitamin C, also known as ascorbic acid, is necessary for the growth, development and repair of all body tissues. It's involved in many body functions, including formation of collagen, absorption of iron, the immune system, wound healing, and the maintenance of cartilage, bones, and teeth.

Vitamin C is one of many antioxidants that can protect against damage caused by harmful molecules called free radicals, as well as toxic chemicals and pollutants like cigarette smoke. Free radicals can build up and contribute to the development of health conditions such as cancer, heart disease, and arthritis.

Thank you to WebMD for that information.

Potassium caught my eye right away, too. That's something I need to limit as a CKD patient, so why would I want to add extra? Maybe if I had a deficiency I would, but this is not usually the case with us. I relied on ***What Is It and How Did I Get It? Early Stage Chronic Kidney Disease*** to remind myself just what this is and why it's important.

One of the electrolytes, important because it counteracts sodium's effect on blood pressure.

This is not looking so good, is it?

Uh-oh, it has 10% of your daily value for sodium… for one serving. Multiply that by three and you get a whopping 30% or 690 mg. of salt/day. Hmmm, I'm only permitted 1500 mg. daily. This accounts for getting close to 50% of my daily sodium allotment.

On mykidney.com {a kidney blog which seems to be defunct now, but does have an image of the ingredient label on this live link.}, Krissi – the writer of the blog – had the following to say about Airborne's Vitamin E content.

If taken as recommended, "Airborne" will provide 300% of the safe daily dose. And like Vitamin A, Vitamin E is also a fat-soluble vitamin and can quickly build up into toxic levels.

However, the 'safe daily dose' for a CKD or ESRD patient is only 8-10mg per day. Just one dose of Airborne actually provides not 300%, but 900% of the safe daily dose for kidney patients.

Back to me here. Notice the herbal ingredients listed at the bottom of the label. What amounts of each are in one dosage? How about in three? And just what do they do to your kidneys? Did you notice that the FDA was in no way involved with this product? And why no clinical studies?

Well, now I know why I can't take Airborne or any other product like it and so do you.

Whoa! Did you know about this?

Airborne Health, a Bonita Springs, Fla.-based herbal supplements firm, has agreed to pay $23.3 million to settle a class-action lawsuit brought against the company for falsely claiming its vitamins prevented colds. Now, let's be fair here. This was back in 2008. Checking into any changes to their formula since then, I could only find changes in their advertising from 'miracle cold cure' to 'immunity booster,' but not for us. We can't handle all the extra bursts of all that good stuff.

Until next year,
Keep living your life!

Index

A

A1C 29-31, 40, 98-9
Airborne 147-9
AKI (Acute Kidney Injury) 94-6
Albumin 41
Anemia, 14
Apps 39

B

Blood
    High Blood Pressure 41, 43-5
    Pressure 83
    Monitoring 106-8
    Sugar 40-2
    Urea 50
    Vessels 41-2
Books
    Kidney Disease: Common Labs and Medical Terminology: The Patient's Perspective (Renal Diet HQ IQ Pre-Dialysis Living) (Volume 4), 6
    Kidney Disease: A Guide for Living, 7
    Living Well with Kidney Disease, 7-8
    Medical Surgical Nursing: Critical Thinking for Collaborative Care, 13
    Understanding Chronic Kidney Disease: A guide for the Non-Specialist, 7
    What You Must Know About Kidney Disease: A Practical Guide to Using Conventional and Complementary Treatments, 8
Brain Fog 49-51
BUN (Blood Urea Nitrogen Test) 50

C

Cholesterol 83
Creatinine 83
Dehydration, 60-1
Depression 16-8
Deviated Septum 46-8
Diabetes 29-30

E

Electrolyte Balance 144-6
EPO (Erythropoietin), 14-5
Exercise, 65-7, 82-4, 113-4

F

Facebook 88-90
Fatigue, 13-5
Food
  Caffeine 105
  Cherries, 68-70
  Eat by Date 34-5
  Fast Food 137-9
  Freezing Food 33-4
  Potatoes, Leeching 54
  Renal Diet 39, 62-4

My Notes:

Have you read my other Chronic Kidney
Disease books?
Available on Amazon.com and B&N.com
(print and digital)
or walk into a B&N to order them.

***What Is It and How Did I Get It?
Early Stage Chronic Kidney Disease***

SlowItDownCKD 2011

SlowItDownCKD 2012

SlowItDownCKD 2013

SlowItDownCKD 2015

SlowItDownCKD 2016

SlowItDownCKD 2017

Follow the blog at
https://gailraegarwood.wordpress.com

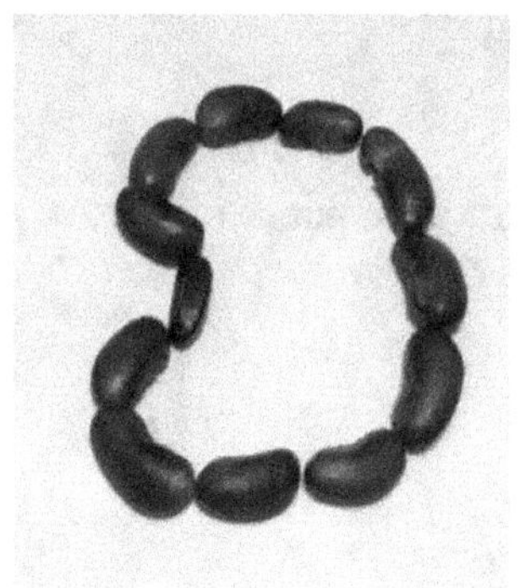

On Instagram, Pinterest, and Twitter go to
@SlowItDownCKD

And then, there's the Facebook page at
*https://www.facebook.com/
SlowItDownCKD/*

Don't forget you can email me at
SlowItDownCKD@gmail.com

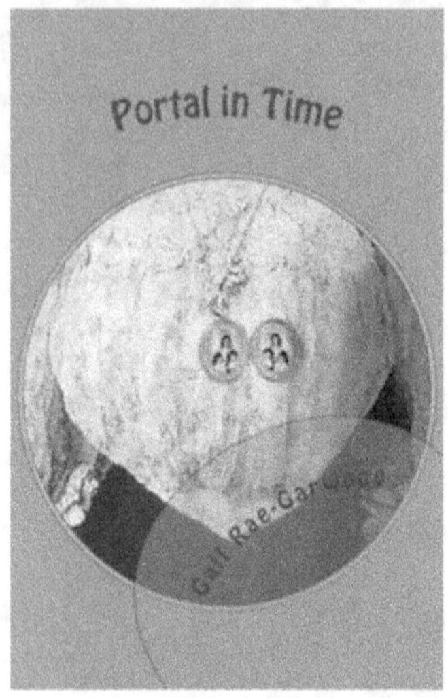

If you'd like to read a time travel romance (above) or fiction based on others' experiences (below), I've written one of each.

www.ingramcontent.com/pod-product-compliance
Lightning Source LLC
Chambersburg PA
CBHW070123260726
48658CB00001B/235